How to Live 100 Years Without Growing Old

Hyaluronic Acid: Nature's Healing Agent

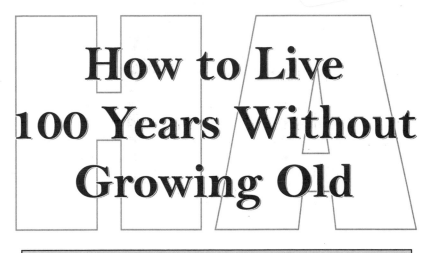

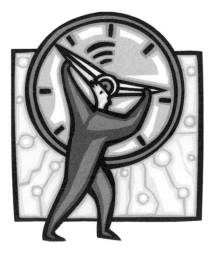

Bill Sardi

Bill Sardi
© Copyright 2002

ISBN 0-9705640-6-6

Accurate indications, adverse reactions, and dosage sched-ules for various products are provided in this book, but it is possible that they may change. The reader is urged to review the package information data of the manufacturers of the food supplements medications mentioned.

The publishers have made every effort to trace the copyright holders for borrowed material. If they have inadvertently overlooked any, they will be pleased to make the necessary arrangements at the first opportunity.

Some images courtesy of ArtToday.com and Photospin.com

Printed in the United States of America
First printing in 2002

Table of Contents

CHAPTER ONE

Was aging reversed in the 1970s?

There are numerous scientific studies that reveal bona fide ways to slow the aging process. Among them are the use of antioxidant food supplements (anti-rusting agents) such as vitamin C, vitamin E and the trace mineral selenium. The daily use of these and other nutrients reduces the risk of age-related changes associated with disease. But what if the cataracts, wrinkles, memory loss and joint pains have already appeared? Now what? Can these aging changes actually be reversed?

Sometimes great medical discoveries are overlooked and as time passes, they are never adopted into the daily practice of modern medicine. Such is the case of Dr. Lester Morrison and his research performed over three decades ago. Dr. Morrison, a California physician, provided case histories of patients who took oral chondroitin sulfate supplements. Here are three astounding case reports.

A 77-year-old retired university professor was seen in 1958. He had a previous heart attack, had atherosclerosis, high blood pressure and enlarged prostate with complaints of overall weakness, pounding heart, skipped heart beats,

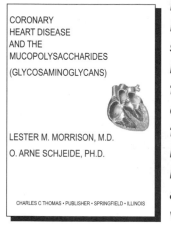

CORONARY
HEART DISEASE
AND THE
MUCOPOLYSACCHARIDES
(GLYCOSAMINOGLYCANS)

LESTER M. MORRISON, M.D.
O. ARNE SCHJEIDE, PH.D.

CHARLES C THOMAS · PUBLISHER · SPRINGFIELD · ILLINOIS

In 1974, Dr. Lester M. Morrison wrote a book showing dramatic improvement in heart function using oral chondroitin sulfate, a food supplement that boosts the production of hyalruonic acid. Other age reversal benefits were also reported.

coldness of extremities, nervousness and insomnia. His blood pressure was 160/100. He was started on 10,000 milligrams a day of chondroitin sulfate. Then after three months this was dropped to 3000 milligrams and finally 1500 milligrams. He had been taking three drugs including Digitalis and nutritional supplements. Within three months of taking the chondroitin sulfate the patient said he "felt wonderful." His fatigue, nervousness and debility had disappeared. The skipped heart beats were no longer reported. His hair began to re-grow and he had dark hair growth replace previous white hair. His prostate gland no longer bothered him and frequent trips to the bathroom at night ceased. His planned prostate removal surgery was cancelled. The urologist said a "remarkable improvement" in his condition had suddenly occurred. His need for prescription drugs waned. There were no side effects. [Morrison LM, Schjeide OA,

Coronary Heart Disease and the Mucopolysaccharides (Glycosaminoglycans), Charles C Thomas, Springfield, Ill, 1974]

A 58-year-old female secretary was seen in 1955. Her heart had enlarged, she had hypothyroidism, osteoarthritis of the back, high cholesterol, chest pain, heart palpitations, nervousness, hot flashes with swollen ankles and puffy skin around the eyes. She was taking thyroid hormone, nitroglycerin, an anti anxiety pill, Premarin, and many other medications and vitamins. She was started on 10,000 milligrams of chondroitin sulfate and 5 months later the dosage was dropped to 2000 milligrams and finally 1500 milligrams per day. On chondroitin sulfate alone she experienced remission of angina chest pain for the first time in over a decade. Within a year the patient had resumed work and had planned to move to Europe now that she was feeling so well. [Morrison LM, Schjeide OA, Coronary Heart Disease and the Mucopolysaccharides (Glycosaminoglycans), Charles C Thomas, Springfield, Ill, 1974]

A 68-year-old retired male was first seen in 1965. He had experienced a previous heart attack (1949), high blood pressure, atherosclerosis, numerous small strokes, visual impairment, exhaustion, inability to walk or stand without assistance, vertigo and fainting.

He had been on blood-pressure lowering drugs, a tranquilizer, other medications and vitamins. Following two months of 10,000 milligrams of chondroitin sulfate supplementation, "striking and dramatic improvement" was noted. All "black outs" and fainting spells ceased. All numbness from previous cerebral accidents disappeared. Vision strikingly improved as did memory, gait, strength and vitality. Patient began walking six miles every day. Hair growth was observed after going bald 15 years previously. New black hair was observed. [Morrison LM, Schjeide OA, Coronary Heart Disease and the Mucopolysaccharides (Glycosaminoglycans), Charles C Thomas, Springfield, Ill, 1974]

These cases of "age reversal therapy" were reported nearly three decades ago by Dr. Lester Morrison. You are likely hearing about them for the first time in this book. Modern medicine has "advanced" to develop more modern therapies that only produce more and more side effects. None compare to Dr. Morrison's documented achievements.

THE VILLAGE OF YUZURIHARA

Dr. Morrison's reports sound similar to an ABC television news report that was aired late in the year 2000. ABC News *Prime Time Live* took their television cameras to the village of Yuzurihara, Japan about an

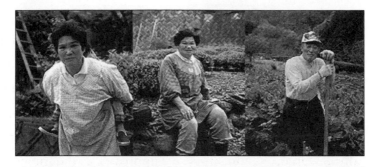

Pictures of the residents of Yuzurihara, Japan continue to astound the world. Yuzurihara has ten times more people living beyond the age of 85 than any community in the United States. Furthermore, these people exhibit youthful skin, flexible joints and good eyesight that is uncharacteristic for their age. Hyaluronic acid has been identified as the molecule responsible for the health and longevity of the residents of Yuzirhara.
Photo courtesy of the East 1999

hour and a half north of Tokyo. The cameras displayed people who defied the clock hands of time. Like Hiroshi Sakamoto who wakes up every morning and farms his fields for four or five hours a day at the age of 86. Sakamoto, who smokes a pack of cigarettes a day, is not unlike others in this village. Tadanao Takahashi, age 93, has soft and smooth skin yet he had worked out in the sun for over 50 years without the use of a sun block. He has the skin of a baby.

Yuzurihara, the "village of long life," has ten times more people who live beyond the age of 85 than any town in the USA and its residents live longer than more

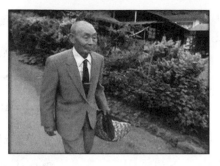

This 86 year old resident of Yuzurihara still works four or five hours a day farming his field. His skin does not show signs of aging even though he smokes a pack and a half of cigarettes daily.   Photo: ABCNews.com

than 900 villages and towns in Japan surveyed by the World Health Organization.

ABC news came to Yuzurihara to discover its anti-aging secret. Dr. Toyosuke Komori, the town doctor, had been studying this population for over 60 years. He noted that there had never been a case of skin cancer in Yuzurihara and one woman in her 90s has flawless skin. Few people developed the age-related health problems of diabetes, heart disease or cancer. Dr. Komori attributed the longevity and good health of the residents of Yuzurihara to a substance called hyaluronic acid. [ABC News Nov. 2, 2000]

What? Hyaluronic acid? Never heard of it! Most people have never heard of hyaluronic acid, not even the people who live in Yuzurihara. The diet in Yuzurihara is different from other parts of Japan. In most of Japan the center of the diet is rice. But in Yuzurihara, which is located on a mountain slope, rice cannot be easily grown and the people eat sticky types of vegetables, particularly a gelatinous root sweet potato-like vegetable

ABC News said, "The residents of Yuzurihara rarely have any reason to see a doctor and they are hardly affected by diseases like cancer, diabetes and Alzheimer's."

called tamaji. Apparently tamaji and other foods helped to maintain high levels of hyaluronic acid throughout the lifetime of these Japanese people.

While we aren't exactly sure which of the foods consumed by the people in Yuzurihara help to maintain healthy HA levels, we are aware of other herbal products that perform similar functions. For example, Echinacea (purple coneflower), an herbal product widely consumed as an immune system stimulator, is known to aid in tissue repair and reduce inflammation in wounds largely by its ability to inhibit hyaluronidase, the enzyme that breaks down HA. Echinacea also stimulates fibroblasts, the cells that rapidly divide in wounds and secrete large quantities of collagen. As Echinacea activates

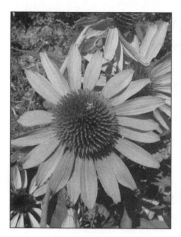

Echinacea, also known as the purple cone flower, is an herb that helps to maintain hyaluronic acid in the human body, thus preventing the spread of infection and tumors.
Photo: Erowid 2002

fibroblasts to produce more HA, this slows the spread of infection in tissues surrounding a wound. [Brodsky J, Echinacea, Continuing Education Module, New Hope Institute, Feb. 1999]

Horse chestnut is another herbal product, often used to treat varicose veins, that works by inhibiting the production of hyaluronidase that degrades hyaluronic acid. [The Lancet 347: 292-94, 1996; Archives Dermatology 134: 1356-60, 1998; BMC Cardiovascular Disorders 1: 5, 2001] All bioflavonoids, found naturally in tea leaves, citrus rind, and the skin of berries, cherries and grapes, inhibit hyaluronidase the breakdown enzyme for HA by virtue of their ability to bind to iron and copper.

The chondroitin sulfate prescribed in the 1970s by Dr. Lester Morrison helps to stimulate the production of hyaluronic acid. It's no wonder that Dr. Morrison's patients reported   astounding reversal of aging.   But over time Dr. Morrison's discovery was forgotten.   It was later categorized as something good for people with heart disease.   Its anti-aging effects were ignored.   Dr. Morrison's former medical institution has completely ignored his achievements.

Since these reports, hyaluronic acid food supplements have been widely marketed here in the USA.   Some of the reports from users are nothing short of remarkable.

A woman, age 43, in Clarkston, Georgia, reports that within weeks the aging lines in her face had decreased and her face looked younger, and remarkably, she could now read fine print in the telephone book without the aid of glasses!

A man in his 50s had a chronic knee condition and had lost enough cartilage so the shoulder on the side of the knee injury had dropped about an inch and he constantly wore a knee brace.   Within five weeks of taking hyaluronic acid food supplements he had abandoned his knee brace and could even resume physical exercise that consisted of walking and trotting again.

A 14-year-old dog, with a painful arthritic knee, could no longer climb the stairs to his second floor bedding and had to be carried up the stairs.   He had been given a pain medication by his veterinarian. Hyaluronic acid was given to the dog to lick off the owner's fingers each morning. The dog began to exhibit a more playful activity level, chasing toys, and running up the stairs again within weeks of being given hyaluronic acid. Pain medication was no longer needed.

Another woman, in her early 50s, began taking hyaluronic acid/chondroitin sulfate supplements to see if it would help her skin. She noticed the fine aging lines in her face were disappearing. But she began noticing other benefits. She had been experiencing hot flashes and night sweats. These subsided with use of the supplement.

A woman in Ohio reports that she took oral hyaluronic acid supplements for four months and noticed the moisture in her skin improved. But she also noticed that HA began to help thicken her hair. She had been battling with thinning hair. Her hair had thinned to the point where others could see her scalp. Her hairdresser noted vast improvement in her hair thinning condition just three months after starting on a course of oral HA therapy.

A Texas couple heard a radio infomercial about HA and decided to try it. They write that others have been approaching them to inquire what they are doing to look so young and healthy. The husband writes, "I can't get over the transition of my wife's looks. My wife is 49 years old and looks better now than most women 10 to 15 years her junior! Her skin as well as mine is very smooth and soft to the touch now." He notes that women have approached him at work in an impromptu fashion to inquire about the changes in his skin texture. He writes: "Lines in our faces have all but disappeared and we have a much healthier look in our faces as well as the rest of our body."

What is hyaluronic acid and chondroitin sulfate? How are these molecules involved in aging? Is humanity upon the threshold of a great discovery?

LETTER FROM A USER OF ORAL HYALURONIC ACID

"I have been taking the formula for approximately four to five months now and have had a lot more energy, have not had any winter or spring colds, and have not had as many blemishes on my face. In fact, my entire skin condition has improved and become much less dry than it was before. But the most astonishing improvement it has made, was in the condition of my hair. As I grew older, my hair became VERY thin—to the point of being able to see my scalp on either side of my head. But in the last month or so, my hair has grown in and has THICKENED. Amazing! I had not been to the beauty shop for three months, and did not say anything to my hairdresser because I wanted to see if she could see any difference, or if it was just my imagination. But when she asked me what I had been putting on my hair to make it thicker, I knew what it had to be. I had not changed any medication, diet, nothing except taking the Ultimate H.A. Formula. She was so impressed that she asked me for some information on the product so she could recommend it to some of her other customers who had very thin hair."

KD
Cincinnati, OH

CHAPTER TWO

Aging: What is it?

How do we know that someone is getting old? What visual cues tell us that someone is old?

British researchers actually conducted a survey to see which physical characteristics were the most common tell-tale signs of aging. Greying of hair, balding and wrinkling of the skin were the most widely reported signs. Arcus senilis, the deposition of cholesterol deposits inside the eyes, observed as a whitish ring on the outside margins of the iris, is also another overt sign of aging.

British researchers report that men who look older than their years have high levels of hemoglobin. Women who appear older than their years had lower than average levels of bilirubin, a substance produced when red blood cells break down. Hemoglobin carries iron while bilirubin is produced upon the breakdown of red blood cells which may release iron. (You'll learn more on the link between iron and aging later.) Thus, these blood tests reveal that iron is a major factor in the visual signs of premature aging. Alcohol use was not correlated with any signs of aging. Smoking was commonly found to

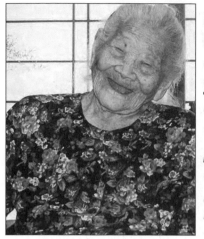

In March of 2002, Kamato Hongo of Japan, at 114 years of age, was declared the world's oldest person by the Guinness Book of Records.
Photo: Agency France-Presse

produce facial wrinkles. [Why Some Age Prematurely, BBC News, Nov. 19, 2001; Bulpitt CJ, Postgraduate Medicine 77: 578-81, 2001]

Slippage and sagging of facial tissue is a telltale sign of aging. Between the ages of 25 and 65 years the nose sags on average by 10 percent, its tip moving downward by a quarter-inch. The brows can sink by a third of an inch, the ears by slightly more, the cheek tissue by as much as a half-inch. Overall, more than 30 percent of a person's facial area may drop from the facial midline to areas below. Crow's feet, sun-caused wrinkles around the temples, is also commonly seen in sunny areas of the world.

The most common signs of aging are balding and graying of the hair, wrinkled skin, stiff joints, need for eyeglasses, and loss of height. All of these signs of aging are attributed to the loss of hyaluronic acid.

Readers need to re-think their definition of aging.

HOW MANY YEARS DO YOU WANT TO LIVE?

Most people, when told they could live longer, to be a hundred, often say they would rather die than live through the ravages of old age. Readers are going to need to re-think their definition of aging. For most people the number of their birthdays is equivalent to their perception of being old and infirm. A rare disease known as progeria will help give us a new understanding of what aging is.

Progeria is a disease where small children appear as they are old, very old. Their skin sags and wrinkles, their hair falls out, they develop blinding cataracts and they don't live long. What is the cause of this premature aging disease? Doctors diagnose progeria by measuring the amount of hyaluronic acid excreted in the urine. Progeria kids excrete 17 times more HA than normal, healthy children. The lesson is clear. The loss of hyaluronic acid is equivalent to aging, not the number of our birthdays. Lose HA and you will look old, regardless of when you were born.

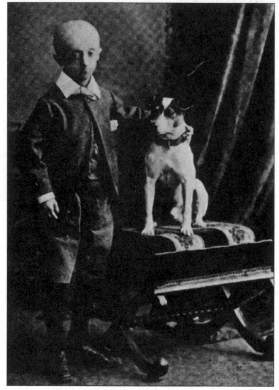

Early photo of young child with progeria,
a disease of premature aging.
Photo: Hastings & Gilford 1911
British Journal of Children's Diseases

The visible signs of aging, wrinkles, stiff joints, diminished eyesight, loss of hair, may have nothing to do with the number of birthdays and everything to do with the loss of hyaluronic acid. Young children with the disease called progeria excrete seventeen times more hyaluronic acid in their urine and appear prematurely old. As the human body ages, there is a slow loss of hyaluronic acid and an accompanying loss of water, which results in loss of support for the skin, jonts and eyes.

WHAT IS HYALURONIC ACID?

By now you may be asking, what is hyaluronic acid and its companion, chondroitin sulfate? These are forms of connective tissue that give substance and form to your body. By binding salt and water, HA expands the space surrounding cells (called the extracellular space). HA is the very glue that keeps your body together. The body is composed of building blocks called cells. In between the cells is collagen or connective tissue, what is sometimes called the ground substance or mortar of the body.

Go to Rome and view an old wall the early Romans built. The bricks are still intact but the mortar has deteriorated. This is because the mortar has dried out and cracked and can no longer support the bricks, so these old walls typically sag in the middle. The lesson here is that the mortar gives way first in a brick wall, not the bricks. The mortar is akin to collagen. When our skin wrinkles, our joints stiffen, and our bodies begin to shrink with old age, we are losing collagen. Or more accurately, the mortar is drying out. For as moisture is lost the collagen (mortar) cracks and can't support the living cells (the bricks).

If the collagen can be kept moist, aging as we know it wouldn't occur. Recognize that the adult human body is about 50-65 percent water, which is roughly 45 quarts. A

CELLS (BRICKS)   COLLAGEN (MORTAR)

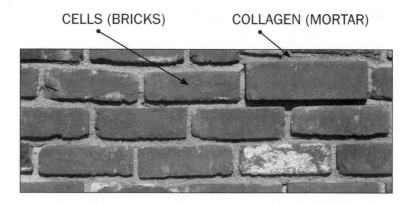

Hyaluronic acid is the "space filler" or support scaffolding for living cells. Living cells are similar to bricks and collagen is akin to mortar that holds the bricks together. Hyaluronic acid keeps the collagen from cracking and drying out. Just 1000 milligrams of hyaluronic acid will hold 6 liters of water.

250-pound adult is carrying about 175 pounds of water. A child's body is approximately 75 percent water and a 3-day old newborn is about 97 percent water. At eight months of age the water content in the body has dropped to 81 percent. About 70 percent of the brain is water, 90 percent of the lungs, 80 percent of blood and 22 percent of bones. And what molecule is holding all that water? The molecule that holds water is hyaluronic acid. HA holds more water than any other molecule and expands by up to 10,000 times its original volume in doing so. One gram of HA can bind up to six liters of water.

AGING IS THE LOSS OF WATER

According to Karl Meyer, the discoverer of hyaluronic acid, the content of HA in body tissues declines in all connective tissues in the course of maturing and aging and thus contributes to the loss of water and consistency of tissues.   [Morrison LM, Schjcide OA, Coronary Heart Disease and the Mucopolysaccharides (Glycosaminoglycans), Charles C Thomas, Springfield, Ill, 1974]

Dr. Fereydoon Batmanghelidj, in his book Your Body's Many Cries For Water (Global Health Solutions 1995), alleges chronic dehydration is the cause of many maladies, including asthma, allergies, arthritis, angina, high blood pressure, diabetes, urinary tract infections, menstrual tension, depression, ulcers and much more. Dr. Batmanghelidj's prescription is for humans to drink an ounce of water for every two pounds (about a kilo) of body weight. A 200-pound person would need to consume about 100 ounces or eight 12-ounce glasses of water a day. Many attest to the simple practice of increasing water consumption to finding a cure for their ailments.

But Dr. Batmanghelidj, searching for a way to hold water in the body and to prevent frequent urination, mistakenly suggests greater consumption of salt.

Americans already consume about 4000 milligrams of sodium a day, more than three times what people in Japan consume where the life span is the highest in the world. Excessive salt consumption can lead to high blood pressure and bone thinning via sodium's competition for absorption with potassium and calcium.

With the long list of ailments remedied by water, modern medicine overlooks the greatest one of all, premature aging, as well as the master water-holding molecule, hyaluronic acid.

The total amount of water in the body decreases with advancing age, and dehydration is common in many diseases. [Journal Nutrition & Aging 1: 142-45, 1997] In older adults the sensation of thirst diminishes and the kidneys are less able to filter water properly. [Geriatric Nursing 21: 84-88, 2000] As little as 2 percent loss of body weight due to dehydration will impair physiological performance. [Journal American Dietetic Assn 99: 200-06, 1999] In a study of dying cancer patients, among whom better than 8 out of 10 who complained of symptoms of dry mouth and thirst, death followed within just two days. [Journal Pain Symptom Management 10: 192-97, 1995] Re-hydration of these terminal patients has up till now proven futile. The patients complain of thirst that water cannot satisfy. That is likely because of the lack of HA.

Hyaluronic acid, or HA, has been called the space filler of the body. It supports or provides scaffolding for all tissues.

WHERE HA IS DISTRIBUTED IN THE BODY:
• 56% IN THE SKIN
• 35% IN THE MUSCLES AND SKELETON
• 9% ELSEWHERE (JOINT FLUID, BLOOD, LYMPH)

MORE THAN JUST GOO

In more recent times researchers have begun to realize HA is more than just goo. It also plays an important role in the way living cells communicate with each other, in the ability of cells to migrate, in wound healing, and in aging. [Journal Clinical Investigation 106: 335-36, 2000] A group of researchers have called HA a "stealth molecule." [Current Opinion in Cell Biology 12: 581-86, 2000]

It's not like the scientific world doesn't know about HA. From 1964 to 2002 there were 8803 research papers published on hyaluronic acid. It's just that the public is being told about HA for the first time. Newsweek magazine published a special edition on breakthroughs in arthritis that included HA injections into knee, shoulder, TMJ and other joints. Anti-wrinkle clinics now tout HA injections performed by dermatologists. For over a decade eye surgeons have been using a form of HA during eye surgery to lubricate instruments and maintain the shape of the eye during cataract surgery. More than 30 million people have received HA treatment. Even more are applying HA in skin creams or using HA eye drops. The HA revolution has begun!

HA = GLUCOSAMINE + GLUCURONIC ACID

Hyaluronic acid is derived from the Greek word for vitreous (hyaloid) and uronic acid.

That's because Karl Meyer first discovered HA in 1934 in the vitreous jelly of the human eye. Readers may be more familiar with one half of its molecular structure, a molecule called glucosamine sulfate which is widely sold as a remedy for arthritis.

HA is a simple negatively-charged sugar-like molecule of alternating molecules of N-acetyl glucosamine and glucuronic acid. The two molecules together are called a disaccharide, that is, two sugar-like molecules linked together. It is a member of what is called the glycosaminoglycan family of collagen molecules. But actually, HA is so special a molecule it should be in a class of its own. Unlike other types of collagen it is not linked to other proteins or sulfur, just water. Growth factors, usually triggered during healing or growth, as well as vitamin C, stimulate the production of collagen but not HA in the skin. [European Journal Biochemistry 173: 261-67, 1988] So HA is a very unusual molecule.

HA should be distinguished apart from collagen. Collagen is a protein that is a component of bone, cartilage and connective tissue. There are many types of collagen, some of them simply described as Type I, Type II, etc. Types I, II, III collagen are the most abundant. In the human body, 90 percent of collagen is Type I collagen. More Type I collagen is found in skin, tendon and bone while more Type II collagen is found in cartilage, spine and the vitreous gel that fills the eye. To reiterate, HA is found within collagen and it supports collagen by virtue of its ability to maintain hydration. HA keeps collagen from cracking, drying out and degrading.

BLOOD LEVELS OF HA

So why not just have a blood test, determine if your HA levels are low and go from there? The problem is that a low circulating level of HA does not necessarily indicate low HA levels in living tissues. In fact, the normal level of HA in the blood circulation is very low, on the order of only millionths of a milligram (nanogram) per milliliter (drop). HA levels must be kept relatively low in the blood circulation because it can cause the viscosity of the blood to change. High HA levels in the blood circulation would likely increase viscosity and make the blood very thick.

Don't be misled by the interpretation of high and low blood levels of HA. The levels of HA in the blood circulation may indicate the body is losing more HA than normal, or that more HA is being produced. Serum HA levels cannot be used to determine adequacy or deficiency. High levels of serum HA are not always desirable. In the healthy adult the HA levels in the blood serum vary between 10 and 100 micrograms per liter. That means circulating levels of HA vary by a factor of ten. Both high serum HA levels and the rate at which HA is excreted in the urine are know to be high in certain disorders, such as liver disease, rheumatoid arthritis, scleroderma and various types of cancer. [Acta Otolaryngology 442: 7-24, 1987; CIBA Foundation Symposium 124: 9-29, 1986] Following major burn injury, HA levels in the blood plasma are known to rise by 5-30 times above normal. [Burns 22: 212-16, 1996]

Loss of HA in the urine could also be a marker of how fast a person is aging. Small children who develop a disease of premature aging called progeria excrete up to 17 times more HA in their urine than normal children.

The serum HA concentration increases with advancing age, which means more HA is being lost. Between

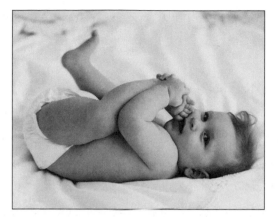

Newborn babies have high levels of
hyaluronic acid in their skin.

Thanks to high levels of hyaluronic acid in their skin,
babies do not develop scars from cuts or scrapes.
Scarless wound healing is a property of hyaluronic acid.

60 and 70 years of age the value is approximately 75 micrograms per liter whereas below age 50 the value is about 30-40 micrograms per liter.

In newborns the concentration of HA in blood serum is around 695 nanograms (1/millionth of a gram) per milliliter but decreases through the first year and then remains relatively constant at about 27 nanograms per milliliter until about the age of 16 years when HA levels in the blood slowly begin to increase with age. But the increase of HA is very gradual till about age 60 when HA levels can exceed 300 nanograms per milliliter. This simply means the body is losing HA at an accelerated rate after age 60. [Cell Physiology 37: C952-57, 1995]

WHERE DOES HA GO ONCE IT IS DEGRADED?

About a third of the hyaluronic acid in the body is degraded and replaced on a daily basis. As HA breaks down it enters the lymph drainage system and makes its way into the blood circulation where it eventually travels to the liver and undergoes digestion and final elimination via the bile fluid. [Cell Physiology 37: C952-57, 1995]

HA concentration in lymph can vary by 250 times. [Biochemistry 236: 521-25, 1986] In cases where limbs swell due to inadequate lymph drainage, it has been found that HA stagnates in the limb which may interfere with lymph drainage, a condition called lymphedema. [Lymphology 31: 173-79, 1998]

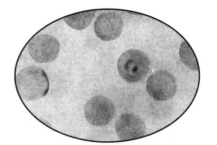

HA is produced throughout the body by cells called fibroblasts.

WHAT DOES HA DO?

OK, OK, you are learning what HA is, but what does it do? Nothing short of magic.

• HA HOLDS WATER IN THE BODY.
• HA ACTS AS A LUBRICANT IN THE HEART VALVES.
• HA IS THE SPONGY SHOCK ABSORBER AT THE ENDS OF BONES.
• HA HOLDS MOST OF THE MOISTURE IN THE SKIN.
• HA MAKES UP 80 PERCENT OF THE HUMAN EYE.
• HA PROVIDES A BARRIER AGAINST THE SPREAD OF INFECTION.
• HA RETARDS THE GROWTH OF CANCER (THOUGH IT HAS A DUAL PERSONALITY IN THIS REGARD).
• HA CAN PRODUCE SCARLESS WOUND HEALING.
• HA HAS ANTIOXIDANT PROPERTIES.
• HA DETOXIFIES THE BODY.
• HA PROVIDES FORM AND SHAPE TO THE BODY.

SIZE IS IMPORTANT

The size, or what is called the molecular weight of HA, is very important. There are three sizes of HA in the human body. In connective tissue and joints HA has a molecular weight of about 4-5 million Daltons. (A Dalton is a measure of the mass of an atom that whirls around a nucleus. Atoms are the smallest particles of matter.)

In lymph fluid HA ranges from 1-2 million Daltons. In blood and cerebrospinal fluid HA has an average molecular weight in the hundreds of thousands. [New Frontiers in Medical Sciences: Redefining Hyaluronan, Elsevier Science, 2000, pp. 7]

An HA molecule could link in a long chain that can reach 10,000 or more double-sugar molecules (called disaccharides) with a molecular mass of around 4 million. The average length of one disaccharide is around 1 nanometer, or 1-millionth of a meter with a molecular weight of around 400 Daltons. That's really small. But it sure can hold a lot of water, 10,000 times it own mass!!

The human body contains about 14,000-16,000 milligrams of HA with about 50 percent of this volume in the skin. Remarkably, about a third of this HA is removed and replaced on a daily basis. [Hascall VC, Laurent TC, Hyaluronan: Structure and Physical Properties, www.glycoforum.gr.jp] Your body is losing and replacing about 3000-4000 milligrams of HA a day.

HOW IS IT MADE?

HA is produced throughout the body by cells called fibroblasts. HA is found inside cells, on the cell surface and as well as in surrounding connective tissue. The rate of HA synthesis is determined by an enzyme (hyaluronan synthase), as well as growth factors, hormones and nutrients. [Acta Otolaryngology 442: 7-24, 1987]

Chondroitin sulfate is a companion to HA. When chondroitin sulfate is administered to rodents intravenously, the levels of HA rise rapidly. Within about an hour HA levels increase by 10-20 times their normal level. [Glycobiology 7: 1209-14, 1997] Various collagens stimulate the production of HA, including dermatan sulfate, glucosamine sulfate and chondroitin sulfate. [Archives Biochemistry Biophysics 240: 146-53, 1985]

HOW MUCH HA IS PRODUCED?

Both collagen and HA rapidly degrade and are replaced in the human body on a daily basis. This means the human body is continually being remolded. Imagine a potter who can keep clay continually moist and remold his vessel perpetually. The normal daily production of hyaluronic acid in man is about 3 to 5 grams, or 3000 to 5000 milligrams. Collagen turnover (old collagen replaced by new collagen) also occurs rapidly, about 3-5 percent per day in many adult tissues and 10% in others. [American Journal Physiology 252: C1-9, 1987] The human body is in a constant state of remodeling and regeneration.

HOW MUCH HA IS LOST DAILY?

Most degraded HA is excreted at the rate of 0.3 to 1.0 micrograms per kilogram (2.2 pounds) of body weight. [CIBA Foundation Symposium, 143: 41-53, 1989] The net daily loss of HA in an adult can vary from 10-150 milligrams of HA. [Am J Respiratory Cell Molecular Biology 23: 431-33, 2000] The daily excretion of HA in adults over age 50 or so is about 150 milligrams. [Clinical Experimental Pharmacology Physiology 11: 17-25, 1984] Oral replacement of HA should be started to put the brakes to aging.

ABOUT CHONDROITIN SULFATE

- Concentrates on the walls of arteries.
- Can be used to treat atherosclerosis.
- Inhibits abnormal blood clotting.
- Concentrates on the valves of the heart.
- Decreases the risk of a heart attack.
- Is a component of cell membranes.
- Is an anti-inflammatory agent.
- Disrupts membranes of some viruses.
- Is a potent antioxidant.
- Concentrates in the bones.
- Rebuilds cartilage.
- Is useful for osteoarthritis.
- Is used to treat neuralgia.
- Lowers oxalate levels and thus reduces the risk of kidney stones.
- Lowers triglycerides (3000 mg per day = 27% reduction).
- Lowers cholesterol (3000 mg per day = 15% reduction).

CHAPTER THREE

Hyaluronidase: The enzyme that breaks down collagen

The human body is undergoing a continual rebuilding process. Night vision cells in the retina undergo partial renewal on a daily basis. Skin cells die off and replace themselves about every 20-30 days. By comparison, brain cells are not shed and replaced like other cells or human would experience an erasure of their memory.

Without breakdown and degradation of some HA every day, undesirable levels of HA would build up in tissues. Fortunately, some HA is broken down at a measured pace by an enzymatic process.

Hyaluronidase is the enzyme that breaks down HA. It is both a good and undesirable enzyme. HA is a polymer, that is, it is linked together in long chains. Hyaluronidase can de-polymerize HA, that is, unzip or unlink it. Hyaluronidase also digests chondroitin sulfate, but at a slower rate than HA. [Matrix Biology 21: 31-37, 2002]

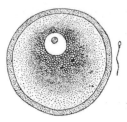 *Hyaluronidase is secreted by human sperm cells to break down the coating around a human ovum (egg).*

Fortunately, there are natural hyaluronidase inhibitors in the body, which are dependent upon magnesium for their full activity, that help maintain HA. Hyaluronidase inhibitor levels in the blood circulation are twice as high in cancer patients. This is probably an attempt by the body to hold on to as much HA as possible.

Hyaluronidase is the same enzyme that is employed by snakes, bees, scorpions and poisonous fish to spread their venom when they sting. While not a venom itself, hyaluronidase aids in the spread of venom. [Experientia 47: 1196-1200, 1991]

Hyaluronidase can be beneficial. For example, hyaluronidase attempts to breakdown HA in cancer so it won't facilitate the spread of tumors. [Matrix Biology 21: 31-37, 2002]

Without hyaluronidase you wouldn't be reading this book. That's because hyaluronidase is secreted by human sperm cells to break down the coating around a human ovum (egg). This facilitates the fertilization of the egg. Without hyaluronidase human life couldn't begin. [Biological Reproduction 56: 1383-89, 1997]

Hyaluronidase is actually a drug (Wydase, Wyeth-Ayerst) that is used as a spreading agent for anesthetics in eye surgery and for other various applications in medicine. It is made from highly purified bovine testicular enzyme. Unfortunately, the sole manufacturer of Wydase has ceased production for various reasons, including the fact its patent has expired and profits are below par. This withdrawal of hyaluronidase is ill timed since researchers are just now beginning to understand some of its therapeutic application. Hyaluronidase could be a potent treatment against cancer. (See the section on cancer below)

WHAT TRIGGERS HYALURONIDASE?

Iron, excess riboflavin, viruses and solar ultraviolet radiation are factors that can accelerate the production of hyaluronidase and the breakdown of HA.

The negative side of hyaluronidase is that it can be used by germs to facilitate the spread of infection and to promote tissue invasion in cancer. [Invasion Metastasis 17: 297-311, 1997]

VIRUSES AND HA

In 1928 a spreading factor that enhances the spread of viruses was discovered which was later identified as hyaluronidase. [Duran-Reynals F, C.R. Society Bulletin 99:6-7, 1928]

It is not surprising that some viruses such as hepatitis B and C and papovirus can produce long-lasting rheumatic symptoms. [American Family Physician 54: 2009-15, 1996] A certain type of encephalitis virus which infects goats can produce progressive symptoms of arthritis. Injecting hyaluronidase into a goat will worsen the disease. [Microbial Pathology 5: 399-406, 1988]

Conversely, HA actually retards the spread of viruses in the joints. [Proceedings Society Experimental Biology Medicine 149: 594-98, 1975]

RIBOFLAVIN AND HA

Riboflavin (vitamin B2) is a photosensitizing vitamin. It turns brown when exposed to sunrays. In living tissues riboflavin enables carbohydrates, proteins and fats to release energy and it is needed for proper growth and reproduction. However, an excess of riboflavin may be harmful, particularly in tissues exposed directly to unfiltered sunlight, such as the skin and eyes.

A lifetime of exposure to unfiltered sunlight combined with excessive riboflavin (vitamin B2) may induce the breakdown of HA in the skin and eyes.

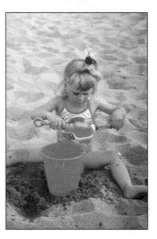

Riboflavin can accelerate skin aging. [Journal Photochemistry Photobiology 14: 105-24, 1992]

Under laboratory conditions, the cornea becomes stiff when bathed in riboflavin and exposed to ultraviolet radiation. Riboflavin however could be utilized in a positive way to treat eye conditions. For example, riboflavin and UV light could be a treatment for keratoconus, a bulging and thinning of the cornea. [Ophthalmologe 94: 902-06, 1997]

Excess riboflavin may produce brown cataracts in the focusing lens of the eyes. [Indian Journal Ophthalmology 46: 233-37, 1998]

Excessive riboflavin and UV light may be harmful to the retina. The exposure of black-eyed rats to ultraviolet radiation whose diet provided excessive amounts of riboflavin resulted in a thinning of the retinal layers. [Experientia 49: 1084-87, 1993]

A lifetime of exposure to unfiltered sunlight combined with excessive riboflavin may induce the breakdown of the vitreous jelly of the eyes. [Current Eye Research 13: 505-12, 1994]

RIBOFLAVIN AND CANCER

Riboflavin, by virtue of its ability to break down HA, could increase or decrease survival in cases of cancer. In the following study, among mice given an anti-cancer drug (Adriamycin), riboflavin alone added to the diet decreased their survivability significantly within a few days. Likewise, when the diet of these animals was deprived of riboflavin, survival was also drastically reduced.

ADRIAMYCIN-TREATED RATS
NORMAL CHOW DIET   SURVIVAL AFTER 12 DAYS = 50%
NORMAL CHOW DIET + RIBOFLAVIN INJECTIONS   SURVIVAL AFTER 20 DAYS = 14%
RIBOFLAVIN-DEFICIENT DIET   SURVIVAL AFTER 5 DAYS = 5%
[PROCEEDINGS EXPERIMENTAL BIOLOGY MEDICINE 188: 495-99, 1988]

The right amount of dietary and supplemental riboflavin is important. Too little riboflavin can also be problematic. Riboflavin deficiency can induce cataracts and reduce the strength of a wound as it heals by decreasing its collagen content. Riboflavin deficiency also impairs growth and may reduce body weight. [Biochemistry Medical Metabolic Biology 42: 185-91, 1989] About 10 milligrams of riboflavin is the suggested upper limit in food supplements. [Proceedings National Academy Sciences 76: 3504-06, 1979]

IRON, COPPER AND HA

Rusting agents like iron and copper can also be troublesome when mixed with riboflavin. The addition of iron to riboflavin further increases the destructive breakdown of HA. [Free Radical Biology Medicine 22: 1139-44, 1997]

Copper is particularly troublesome in the vitreous jelly of the eyes and can cause this jelly to turn to liquid quite readily. [Ophthalmic Research 29: 37-41, 1997]

Iron is an essential mineral required for the production of oxygen-carrying hemoglobin in red blood cells. Iron can become uncontrolled and turn into a rusting agent when it is unbound from proteins that keep it in check. Free, unbound iron generates free radicals that encourage the production of hyaluronidase that can destroy HA. Vitamin C can convert iron into a more toxic form. Ascorbic acid (vitamin C) when combined with iron also accelerates degradation of the vitreous gel of the human eye. [Ophthalmic Research 24: 1-7, 1992] Both copper and iron, when unbound to proteins (called free copper and free iron), can break down the vitreous jelly of the eyes.

METAL CHELATORS

There are numerous agents, both drugs and herbal bioflavonoid compounds found in citrus fruits and berries, as well as molecules found in whole grains and seeds, that can bind to iron, copper and other potentially toxic metals. These are called metal chelators. Once bound, these metals are rendered harmless and make their exit via the human circulatory system to the kidneys and bladder.

By virtue of their iron-binding quality, bioflavonoids inhibit the production of hyaluronidase. When HA and antioxidants are combined in skin tissue there is a slight reduction in the breakdown of HA. But when iron or copper chelators (removers) are added, the breakdown of HA is reduced by 3-4 times. [Free Radical Biology Medicine 23: 996-1001, 1997]

Many other hyaluronidase inhibitors are found in nature. Some natural hyaluronidase inhibitors are curcumins from the spice cumin, glycyrrhizin from licorice, tea leaves, and hydrangenols from hydrangea. [Matrix Biology 21: 31-37, 2002; Biol Pharm Bulletin 20: 973-77, 1997] Bioflavonoids found in parsley and chamomile (apigenin), artichoke, basil and celery (luteolin), and in strawberries, leeks, kale, broccoli, limes, asparagus (kaempferol) have been found to inhibit the activity of hyaluronidase. [Experientia 47: 1196-200, 1991]

Bioflavonoids are effective against viruses. In a laboratory dish it can be observed that bioflavonoids inhibit viruses while the addition of hyaluronidase abolishes this protection. [Arzneimittelforschung 28: 347-50, 1978]

Bioflavonoids inhibit the activity of hyaluronidase in sperm. [Biological Reproduction 56: 1383-89, 1997] It is possible that a strong bioflavonoid by virtue of its ability to inhibit hyaluronidase would make a natural anti-conception agent since hyaluronidase is required for sperm to break through the lining of the ovum to fertilize a human egg.

Since hyaluronidase is secreted in snake and insect venom, survival time is prolonged in rodents given bioflavonoids prior to injection of poisonous snake venom. [Experientia 47: 1196-1200, 1991; Experientia 47: 1196-2000, 1991]

Milk thistle, traditionally used in herbal medicine, is a potent inhibitor of hyaluronidase. [Biochemical Pharmacology 40: 397-401, 1990]

In a study of four different bioflavonoids, quercetin was found to be a superior inhibitor of hyaluronidase. [Biological Reproduction 56: 1383-89, 1997]

THE ATTACK OF THE OXYGEN FREE RADICALS

Free radicals, atoms that are on a mission to obtain a missing electron, break down HA while antioxidants preserve HA. A particular type of internal rusting agent called super oxide, produced naturally in the body, readily breaks down HA. There is a very close relationship between the provision of iron and the development of super oxide. [Inflammation 10: 15-30, 1986]

Phagocytes, special immune cells in the blood circulation, can react with iron to form another rusting agent called the hydroxyl radical which attacks HA. [Clinical Science 64: 649-53, 1983]

CHAPTER FOUR

Too much HA

Can you have too much collagen? Yes you can. There are disorders where there is excessive buildup of HA.

Actually, a deficiency of hyaluronidase can produce developmental problems in children who are of short stature, mentally retarded, and exhibit other problems. One of these disorders is Gaucher's Type I disease which has responded to enzyme replacement therapy (glucocerebrosidase). So some researchers believe the provision of the enzyme hyaluronidase to people with collagen storage disorders may be beneficial. [New England Journal Medicine 335: 1029-33, 1996; Science 256: 794-99, 1992]

If there is an example of excess HA it is in a wrinkled Chinese dog called the shar pei. Shar pei dogs have much higher levels of HA in their skin, which is the reason for their unique skin folds. HA in the blood plasma of shar pei dogs ranges from 93-918 micrograms per liter whereas other types of dogs the HA concentration ranges from 25-321 micrograms per liter. The case of a human baby born with excess HA accumulation in the skin has

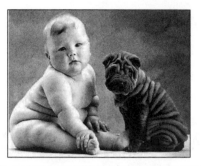

Young children have high amounts of hyaluronic acid in their skin, which results in scarless wound healing. Sharpei dogs also exhibit high amounts of HA, which results in the characteristic folds in their skin.
Photo: Photos Bizarres at Le Site De Dominique

been reported, which dissipated by the age of three. Hyaluronidase levels were normal. [Journal Pediatrics 136: 62-68, 2000]

Localized accumulation of HA occurs in several human diseases such as sarcoidosis, lung fibrosis, farmer's lung, organ rejection, heart attack and human inflammatory bowel diseases. A transient buildup of HA occurs in wound healing. [Journal Internal Medicine 242: 49-55, 1997]

On a temporary basis, more HA is produced during healing. Patients in shock, with burns and septicemia, rapidly produce HA. [Matrix Biology 21: 31-37, 2002]

Conditions where elevated serum HA levels have been reported:

• Rheumatoid arthritis

• Scleroderma

• Psoriatic arthritis

• Psoriasis

• Malignancies

• Liver disease

[The Biology of Hyaluronan, CIBA Foundation Symposium 143, John Wiley & Sons, 1989, p. 233-47]

FIBROSIS (SCARRING)

Fibrosis refers to scar tissue buildup.

An estimated 45 percent of deaths are attributed to scarring or fibrosing diseases. The human body responds to trauma by scarring. Fibrosis is excessive scarring instead of normal wound healing. Trauma, surgery, infection, burns, radiation, alcohol and toxins may promote fibrosis. Alcoholic liver disease is characterized by fibrosis. Excessive production of Type I collagen is often seen in lung diseases. Scar tissue that forms following a heart attack is an example of fibrosis, which impairs the ability of the heart to pump. [Journal Intl Medical Research 6: 217-26, 1978]

Scleroderma, keloids and atherosclerosis are other examples of fibrosing diseases. Drugs, such as Fibrogen's P4H, inhibit fibrosis and in one clinical trial reduced mortality from 39 percent to 9 percent following a heart attack. Fibrosis impairs the ability of the heart to pump and may lead to congestive heart failure. Approximately 400,000 new cases of congestive heart failure are reported each year. [Fibrogen Press release, November 15, 2000]

Fibrosis is associated with iron and copper overload (hemochromatosis and Wilson's disease). Chemicals and drugs such as alcohol, cancer drugs like methotrexate and other chemical agents promote fibrosis. Fibrosis appears to be controlled by proteins produced in the liver that bind to iron such as ferritin and transferrin.

Normally a little bit of new collagen is being made to replace small amounts that have broken down. But in some instances too much collagen may accumulate. This is what happens in a condition called scleroderma. In scleroderma collagen is produced as if there were some kind of perpetual wound healing going on. Joints and lungs don't work well because there is a buildup of collagen. Scleroderma means "thick skin" and the disease can solely affect the skin or the skin and internal organs. It is characterized by narrowed blood vessels and sensitivity to cold in the fingertips. Scleroderma is categorized as an autoimmune disorder.

Too much HA can also develop among patients with cystic fibrosis. Cystic fibrosis patients often develop liver problems. Among young cystic fibrosis patients who have no evidence of liver disease, their HA levels have been found to be normal. Cystic fibrosis patients who have liver disease exhibit about four times more HA concentration in their blood serum. There is no correlation between lung function and HA concentration, suggesting an inability of the liver to clear HA rather than overproduction locally in the lung. Elevated serum HA levels may serve as a marker to indicate which cystic fibrosis patients will develop liver problems. [Archives Diseases Childhood 86: 190-93, 2002]

Since fibrosis frequently occurs in the lung in pulmonary fibrosis or scleroderma, certain supplemental nutrients that inhibit fibrosis may be employed.

Taurine, an amino acid, stimulates collagen formation and retards fibrosis. [Biochemistry Pharmacology 62: 1107-11, 2001] Both taurine and niacin (vitamin B3) have been shown to block lung fibrosis. [Journal Pharmacology Experimental Therapeutics 293: 82-90, 2000] In animals, taurine and niacin almost completely prevent chemically-induced lung fibrosis. [Advances

Taurine, an amino acid, and niacin, a B vitamin, help to retard fibrosis (scarring).

Experimental Medicine Biology 315: 329-40, 1992] Researchers indicate niacin and taurine "have great therapeutic potential in the intervention of the development of fibrosis in animals and humans." [Environmental Health Perspectives 102: 137-47, 1994] Taurine and niacin apparently inhibit the production of Type I and III collagen. [Journal Pharmacology Experimental Therapy 277: 1152-57, 1996] Antioxidants, such as N-acetyl cysteine, may also help to inhibit fibrosis in the lung. [European Respiratory Journal 17: 1228-35, 2001]

Undesirable free radicals induce something called growth factor-beta 1 (TGF-beta 1) which then promotes the deposition of Type I and IV collagen into tissues like the kidneys. The kidneys then stiffen and blood pressure rises. Conventional medicine uses angiotension converting enzyme inhibitors (ACE inhibitors) to stop this process of fibrosis. However, oral taurine supplements have been shown to completely block increases in Type I and IV collagen and prevent kidney fibrosis in animals. [American Journal Renal Physiology 278: F122-29, 2000]

Taurine also works to inhibit the aggregation of blood platelets that form blood clots. In humans taking 400-700 mg of taurine, blood resists platelet aggregation by 30-70 percent. [American Journal Clinical Nutrition 49: 1211-16, 1989]

Since HA is highly concentrated in the skin, joints and eyes, the following chapters will concentrate on these topics.

TESTIMONY OF BIOCELL COLLAGEN II USER
MENOPAUSE SYMPTOMS SUBSIDE

I have taken the BioCell Collagen II formula since mid-December. I expected to wait for six months before I would see any results. However, I began seeing improvements in my health which I believe are directly related to this product, which occurred before that time period was up.

I had been experiencing hot flashes and night sweats. After 4 weeks of taking the HA formula I found I was experiencing milder and less frequent instances of either hot flashes or night sweats. I continued to improve and now virtually have no problem. I feel this information may be of benefit to other menopausal women.

CHL
Bethlehem, PA
March 27, 2002

CHAPTER FIVE

HA and the Skin

Remarkable, youthful changes in the skin are reported and observed among individuals who take HA supplements.

The average human lifespan has increased considerably in developed countries so that aging skin is a problem experienced by a greater proportion of the population. Treatments include skin creams and topical preparations including glycolic acid, chemical peels, botulinum injections, collagen and HA injections, dermabrasion and laser resurfacing in the treatment of wrinkles. [Schewiz Med Wochenschr 150: 1272-78, 2000]

More than half of the HA in the body is in the skin. It's no wonder, since skin is renewed more readily than many other tissues in the body and it is exposed to trauma, solar radiation, heat, pressure and other assaults. So it needs continual renewal. Human skin is made up of billions of cells, 9.5 million to the square inch. A few billion of these are shed each day as old skin cells die off and new ones replace them. Between the ages of 15 and 25 years the skin renews itself about every 20 days, but this increases to about every 28 days as humans age.

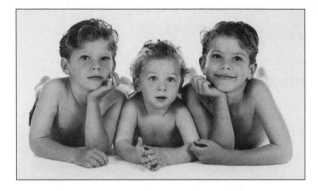

Human skin is 72 percent water. The loss of even 2 to 4 percent of water from the skin produces dryness and wrinkling. Youthful skin is rich in hyaluronic acid (HA). The slow, progressive loss of HA with advancing years produces skin that appears aged.

Human skin is 72 percent water. About 4 percent of the body's water is lost through the skin each day. Most of that water is being held by HA. The loss of water content in the skin results in wrinkles. There is a progressive loss of HA in aging skin. This accounts for the striking appearance of aged skin, wrinkling, and diminished elasticity. [Int J Dermatology 33: 119-22, 1994]

Skin aging is accelerated by exposure to solar ultraviolet radiation, hormonal changes in women and other aging changes in the body. By far the most serious of these aging factors is sunlight. With aging the skin becomes itchy, wrinkled, rough and dry. By the seventh decade of life most people have at least one skin disorder.

Compare aged skin to that of a baby. The dermis of people over age 60 often contains zero HA. The infant's skin is loaded with hyaluronic acid. In babies, any cuts or scrapes heal without scarring because of the high HA content. This is the ideal state of the skin and it never returns as humans leave infancy.

The amniotic fluid that surrounds a developing baby inside a woman is seawater-like fluid that is rich in hyaluronic acid. Any surgery performed in the first or second trimester on an unborn child will not produce scarring. Scarless wound healing has been observed in fetal surgery and is due to the high concentrations of HA in the fetus. [New Frontiers in Medical Sciences: Redefining Hyaluronan, Elsevier Science, 2000, p. 289-96] In adults, skin heals, but the repair may produce fibrosis (scarring) and sometimes contracture. In adult wound healing there is a rapid increase in HA for 3 days and by day 7 there is no detectable HA. Instead, other types of collagen take over.

The rapid production of HA by fibroblast cells in the early states of wound healing result in brisker healing and reduced scarring. [Medical Hypotheses 47: 273-75, 1996]

ESTROGEN AND THE SKIN

Women who take estrogen replacement hormone therapy during menopause often report that their skin feels better. It's no surprise. Estrogen encourages the production of HA in the skin, while progesterone inhibits HA production. [J Invest Derm 87: 668-73, 1986] To prove this in a laboratory study, cells from the human uterine cervix were incubated with glucosamine and then exposed to various hormones. Progesterone suppressed HA production by 22 percent, and DHEA, a hormonal precursor for estrogen, enhanced it by 22 percent. Estrogen enhanced HA production by 12 percent. Progesterone appears to breakdown high-molecular weight HA into lower-molecular weight fragments. [FEBS Letters 402: 223-26, 1997]

In rodents, the administration of estrogen elevates the production of HA in breast tissue. Progesterone, administered alone, only elevates chondroitin sulfate. When both hormones were administered, all of the forms of collagen are elevated. [Acta Physiolog Scandinavia 168: 385-92, 2000]

Estrogen has long been known to have a positive influence upon skin by preventing skin aging. Topical and oral use of estrogen can increase skin collagen content and moisture. Estrogen accomplishes this in part

Estrogen helps to maintain skin moisture. A decline in estrogen levels results in dryness of skin.

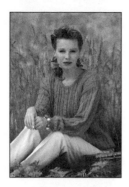

by raising HA levels in the skin. [Clinical Dermatology 2: 143-50, 2001] Some experimental studies show that estrogen improves water content, HA and collagen via stimulation of the fibroblast cells. Skin thickness can be increased by 10-20 percent in treated women. [Therapie 51: 67-70, 1996] Anti-estrogens like Tamoxifen and soy-phytoestrogens appear to block the production of HA in the skin. [Biochim Biophys Acta 627: 199-206, 1980]

HA AND ANTI-INFLAMMMATORY AGENTS

The use of a non-steroidal anti-inflammatory agent (Diclofenac-Voltaren) with hyaluronic acid has been successfully used to treat solar aged skin (actinic keratosis). A clinical cure (resolution of all skin lesions) was achieved in 47 percent of subjects treated compared with 19 percent of patients treated with an inactive placebo. [Drugs Aging 14: 313-19, 1999]

VITAMINS, HA AND THE SKIN

In 1978 Japanese researchers injected two B vitamins, pantothenic acid and vitamin B6, into the skin of mice. The high-dose vitamin injection significantly increased HA concentration in the skin. These researchers theorized one of the mechanisms involved is the estrogen-like effect of vitamin B6. [Journal Nutrition Science Vitaminology 24: 589-91, 1978]

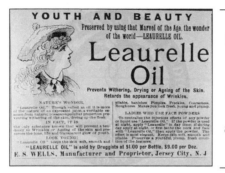

Dryness of the skin, hair, eyes and nails is common among women over age 40. For centuries, women have applied various agents to their skin to retain moisture.

HA SKIN TREATMENTS

HA injections at anti-wrinkle clinics are now becoming popular. Pure HA (Restylane and Juvederm) are also injected by physicians to reduce fine lines and superficial defects. [Aesthetic Plastic Surgery 25: 249-55, 2001] DermaLive is a long-term anti-wrinkle reduction product composed of hyaluronic acid produced from a non-animal source (cell culture) combined with an acrylic hydrogel. The product was first marketed in France and then the rest of Europe beginning in 1998. It is used to treat skin depressions, create volume for lips and sunken cheekbones, and provides a good alternative to other implantable materials. Two to three injections are required to bring about reduction of wrinkles or other defects. [Aesthetic Plastic Surgery 25: 249-55, 2001] About 80 percent of HA injections produce satisfying results. [Dermatological Surgery 24: 1317-25, 1998]

Dermatologists apply glycolic acid (alpha hydroxyl acids) to improve sun-damage skin. It is interesting to note that the application of glycolic acid elevates hyaluronic acid in the dermis and epidermis. [Dermatological Surgery 27: 429-33, 2001]

HA AND VITAMIN A

In mice, skin exposed to fast-tanning ultraviolet-B radiation loses HA, but there is a marked increase in HA when topical vitamin A (all-trans retinoic acid) is applied after exposure to UV rays. [J Investigative Derm 106: 505-09, 1996]

Retinoic acid, a form of vitamin A, stimulates the incorporation of glucosamine into HA which then boosts keratinocytes to produce HA in the epidermis of the skin. [Journal Investigative Dermatology 92: 326-32, 1989]

HA AND VITAMIN D

Vitamin D plays a role in the regulation of HA. HA is redistributed in chicks that are deficient in vitamin D. [Bone 18: 429-35, 1996] Vitamin D is a regulator of skin cells, the keratinocytes, fibroblasts and adipocytes. Solar radiation can cause a disappearance of adipocytes (fatty cells) and an accumulation of collagen such as HA and chondroitin. Application of vitamin D to the skin prevents the disappearance of adipocytes and the accumulation of collagen, which results in an anti-wrinkling effect. [Toxicology Applied Pharmacology 173: 99-104, 2001]

HA AND VITAMIN C IN THE SKIN

Vitamin C is now widely used in anti-aging skin creams. Vitamin C stimulates collagen formation in skin fibroblasts but does not have an effect upon HA. [Eur J Biochem 173: 679, 1988] One study indicates Vitamin C reduces HA production in skin. [J Cell Science 64: 245-54, 1983]

HA AND SCLEROSIS

Scleroderma patients suffer from excessive HA in the skin. In one study the serum HA levels were 131 micrograms per liter in sclerosis patients versus 49

HUMAN SKIN LAYERS

Epidermis

Dermis

Hypodermis

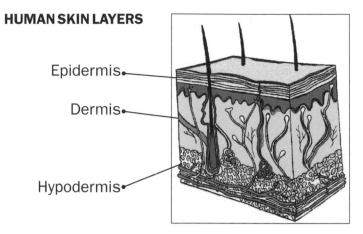

micrograms per liter in healthy patients. [Ann Rheum Disease 44: 614-20, 1985] In scleroderma, the skin's fibroblast cells produce more HA than normal cells. [Arthritis Rheum 27: 1040-45, 1984]

HA AND PSORIASIS

In psoriasis the skin is renewing itself at an accelerated rate. Instead of renewal taking 30 days it takes just three or four. This produces skin that is inflamed, red, dry and scaly. Psoriasis plaque is composed of an accumulation of several layers of dead skin. The serum levels of HA are elevated by 3 times in patients with psoriasis and rheumatoid arthritis compared to health individuals. [Clinical Rheumatology 19: 455-57, 2000] This means in psoriasis the HA in the skin is being regenerated so fast that undue high amounts of used-up HA are being eliminated via the blood circulation. If this is so, then possibly viruses may be involved in initiating psoriatic

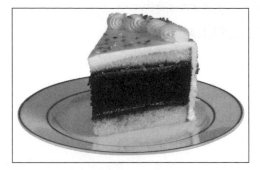

Recipe for Moisture:
Just as a cake recipe calls for the addition of oil to produce a moist cake, humans require oil to hold moisture in the skin.

skin problems since viruses cause a rapid breakdown of HA. Various studies show there is a connection between viral infections and psoriasis. [Archives Dermatology 137: Oct. 2001; European Journal Dermatology 12: 75-76, 2002] Therefore, nutrients that helps fight viruses and also help to maintain HA should be helpful in cases of psoriasis. This is exactly what is found. Bioflavonoids obtained from the bark of the French maritime pine tree are considered to be beneficial for patients with psoriasis. [Phytotherapy Research 15: 76-78, 2001] The addition of folic acid, a B vitamin, iron and protein to the diet has thrown psoriasis into remission in some instances. [International Journal Dermatology 32: 582-86, 1993]

ANOTHER CAUSE OF DRYNESS:
LACK OF ESSENTIAL FATS

There is another essential nutrient, other than HA, that helps retain moisture in the body and it should be mentioned before this book progresses any further. Many readers, particularly females, who experience symptoms of dryness, will read this book with interest. Just as it has been stated in this book that HA holds water, so do the essential fats help to retain water.

Just as a cake recipe calls for the addition of oil to produce a moist cake, humans require oil to hold moisture. Living cells are filled with water which is held inside by a fatty outside membrane. Since water and oil don't mix, oils in the body are a natural way of holding moisture.

Dry skin, dry hair, dry eyes (redness, itching, burning eyes), brittle nails, dry mouth (Sjogrens' syndrome), are all common symptoms experienced by females over the age of 40. Hormonal changes are often the underlying causes of these symptoms. These symptoms of dryness may also be induced by a lack of essential fatty acids. Fats are also required in order to produce hormones.

The moisturizing oils usually added to the diet that encourage moisture retention are evening primrose oil, borage oil and black currant seed oil. These are available as food supplements at health food stores.

These good fats really work. Fatty acids have been shown to increase the time it takes for tears to evaporate from the surface of the eyes. [Rheumatoid Arthritis 4: 165-67, 1984] Essential fatty acids, vitamin C and vitamin B6 have been shown to be successful in restoring normal tear secretion rates to the surface of the eyes. [Medical Hypotheses 6: 225-32, 1980]

Rheumatoid arthritis patients often experience symptoms of dryness. The essential oils from evening primrose, borage or black currant seed have been used successfully to reduce symptoms of joint pain in both rheumatoid and osteoarthritis. [British Journal Nutrition 85: 251-69, 2001]

To name a few good brands, products like Cod Liver Oil Skin Formula made by Twinlab, which provides cod liver oil, flaxseed (linseed) oil and black currant seed oil, or Barlean's Omega Twin which provides borage and flaxseed oil, are excellent in regards to relieving symptoms of dryness. A remarkable new product, Purity's Internal Rejuvenation Formula, combines the moisturizing fatty acids from borage and cod liver oil with hyaluronic acid. It also contains natural sunscreens (beta carotene, ferulic acid) to protect skin from solar radiation.

PLASTIC SURGERY IN A BOTTLE?

"I am a Certified Orofacial Myologist, specializing in facial muscles. I work with orthodontists, dentists, plastic surgeons, dermatologists, chiropractors, etc., who refer patients to me for various facial problems, and I teach 'non-surgical face life' classes, as well. I heard of hyaluronic acid on a radio news broadcast and began a clinical study of its benefits in July of 2001. Since we take before and after photos of all of our clients, these pictures would serve as evidence of any age reversal properties for hyaluronic acid (elimination of fine lines and wrinkles). By the end of 2001, I was ready to report on the results of using oral HA on my patients and myself. I see definite changes in the nasal-labial folds in all our faces and a noticeable smoothness in our facial skin that is softer and definitely more youthful! My husband has also noticed some smoothness as well. I submit these photos as proof of the age reversal properties of oral hyaluronic acid and facial muscle toning exercise."

Sandra R. Coulson
Denver, Colorado

Sandra R. Coulson & Associates, Inc.
2121 South Oneida Street, Suite #633
Denver, CO 80224
Phone: 303-759-2760 Fax: 303-759-2971
www.srcoulson.com

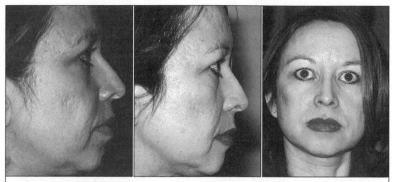

01-06-02   04-09-02   06-25-02

Three months on oral HA (BioCell Collagen II™). Notice the indentation on the cheeks and lip areas, which are filled in just months
later. Almost 6 months on oral HA (front 6/25/02). Dissapear-
ance of indentation in the nasal area and lips noted.

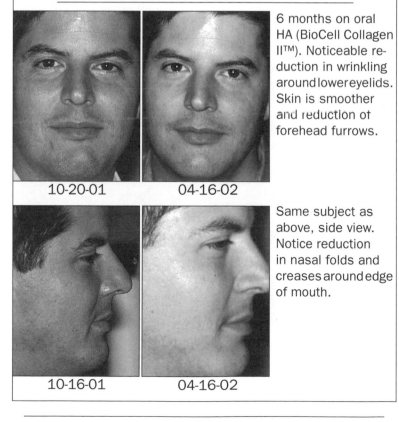

6 months on oral
HA (BioCell Collagen
II™). Noticeable re-
duction in wrinkling
around lower eyelids.
Skin is smoother
and reduction of
forehead furrows.

10-20-01   04-16-02

Same subject as
above, side view.
Notice reduction
in nasal folds and
creases around edge
of mouth.

10-16-01   04-16-02

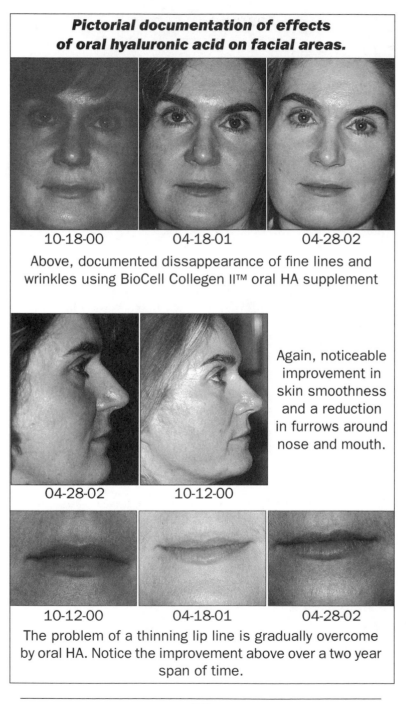

Pictorial documentation of effects of oral hyaluronic acid on facial areas.

10-18-00   04-18-01   04-28-02

Above, documented dissappearance of fine lines and wrinkles using BioCell Collegen II™ oral HA supplement

04-28-02   10-12-00

Again, noticeable improvement in skin smoothness and a reduction in furrows around nose and mouth.

10-12-00   04-18-01   04-28-02

The problem of a thinning lip line is gradually overcome by oral HA. Notice the improvement above over a two year span of time.

Testimony Letter

April 30, 2002

Sandra Coulson
Sandra Coulson & Associates
2121 South Oneida St., Suite 633
Denver, CO 80234

Dear Mrs. Coulson

I am writing this to tell you how happy I am with a product that you asked me to trial for you. That is Purity's Ultimate H.A. Formula.

I have been using the product for about 7 months now and am delighted with the results I am seeing. I have been consistently using 3 tablets a day (before a meal). Within the first two weeks, I noticed improvement in the skin on my face. Tiny wrinkles seemed lessened and the texture smoother. Two work associates (Laura and Bob, both patients of yours) asked me what I was doing during that first month because my skin looked nicer.

I have also noticed that cellulite is noticeably reduced.

This product, combined with the terrific facial exercises you have taught me, is giving me a much more youthful appearance. Another work associate (Jim) was shocked to find out I was 10 years older than he had assumed. I attribute this completely to the facial exercise regimen and the Ultimate H.A. formula.

Thanks so much,

Darlinda

Darlinda Coe

LETTER FROM A USER OF BIOCELL COLLAGEN II™

I just wanted to let you know how I really enjoy the BioCell Collagen II™ HA formula. When I first started to take them, I began to wonder if they were working. Then it hit me about a month later, they were working because I used to be bothered by my wrists and hands falling asleep due to carpal tunnel. Not any more! I do a lot of gardening for fun and I can do it now without being annoyed by a wrist problem. Thanks again!

CH
June 28, 2002

CHAPTER SIX

HA and the Joints

HA is a major factor, if not the most important factor, in arthritis. In joints, the joint (synovial) fluid is attacked by free radicals, degraded (depolymerized) and the joint loses its lubrication. Friction occurs and the joint degenerates. The addition of HA to joints reduces joint friction. [Clinical Biomechanics 12: 246-52, 1997] Glucosamine and chondroitin sulfate stimulate HA production in joint fluid. [Medical Hypotheses 54: 798-802, 2000]

The most pressing need is the development of a non-surgical treatment to relieve symptoms of osteoarthritis that can improve function and stop its progression. [Clinical Orthopedics 385: 36-45, 2001] It has been recommended that treatments for osteoarthritis focus on the synovial fluid inside the joint capsule. [Medical Hypotheses 54: 798-802, 2000] The replenishment of HA to joint tissues is based on the concept that a normal physiological component of synovial fluid is being used. [Am J Orthopedics 29: 80-88, 2000] In synovial fluid, HA acts as an antioxidant. [Arthritis Rheumatology 31: 63-71, 1988] HA is also a natural anti-inflammatory agent. [Agents Actions 43: 44-47, 1994] HA is an

LETTER FROM A USER OF ORAL HYALURONIC ACID (BIOCELL COLLAGEN II™)

"I recently started taking hyaluronic acid and would just like to say how great it's working for me. I've been a self-employed piano mover for the last ten years and have been having major problems with my knees from all the years of extremely heavy lifting. I'm only 32 years old and was in fear that I was getting close to knee surgery, and the end of my business/career as a mover. I was having trouble and pain from simply standing and walking. I was in fear every day that my knees were gonna blow out while on the job and my income would be over. I heard about the HA product on the radio about a month ago and have only been taking them for about two weeks. What I can't believe is that the pain in both my knees is completely gone! I get up...No pain...I work all day...No pain. We even moved a grand piano upstairs to a second floor this week, which I thought I would suffer for, and it didn't bother me a bit.

I don't know if it's some kind of coincidence, but for whatever reason, my pain is gone and my future's looking up. The problem had been increasing for abou thte last six to eight months, and within two weeks of taking HA...it's gone! Thanks a million."

LG

anti-inflammatory agent and pain reliever in joints. [Medical Hypotheses 50: 507-10, 1998] Glucosamine and chondroitin sulfate stimulate HA production in joint fluid. [Medical Hypotheses 54: 798-802, 2000; 50: 507-10, 1998]

Doctors are injecting HA every day into arthritis joints and reporting successful results. Could HA be the cure for arthritis that millions have been waiting for?

Newsweek magazine's special issue on arthritis announced on September 3, 2001 that synthetic HA injected into arthritic joints can provide relief from pain and stiffness. The series of injections cost about $1200. [Newsweek, September 28, 2001]

The January 2002 issue of Consumer Reports indicated there is sufficient evidence that products containing chondroitin sulfate and/or glucosamine sulfate, in adequate amounts, can ease arthritis symptoms. Generally, 1500 milligrams of glucosamine and 1200 milligrams of chondroitin sulfate are reported to produce results.

In January of 2001 a landmark study was published in The Lancet, a prestigious British medical journal. It was a surprising study since a wide array of prescription drugs are available to treat arthritis, but a nutritional product gained attention. As noted in Lancet, "it came from an unexpected quarter." It wasn't a prescription drug. It was an over-the-counter remedy. The three-year study suggests that glucosamine sulfate retards the progression of symptomatic knee arthritis. Lay aside the issue of pain for a moment. Glucosamine was slowing down the progression of the disease itself.

Dr. Tim McAlindon wrote then "it is time for the profession to accommodate the possibility that many nutritional products may have valuable therapeutic effects and to regain the credibility of the public at large." [The Lancet 357: January 2001; 357: 251-56, 2001]

It may come as a surprise to learn that 7 in 10 people over the age of 50, and virtually everyone over age 70 have osteoarthritis and modern medicine's cupboard of cures is empty. All that modern medicine can offer for osteoarthritis is the relief of pain and stiffness. Pain relievers don't address the cause of the disease, which is the loss of HA in the lubricating synovial fluid between the joints with advancing age.

For clarification, osteoarthritis is the common form that affects 95 percent of arthritis sufferers. It is the wear-and-tear type of arthritis. Rheumatoid arthritis only affects about 3 percent of the adult population and is the autoimmune form of the disease. There are many other forms of arthritis including gouty, psoriatic and infectious, but the osteo and rheumatoid varieties make up most of the cases.

Osteoarthritis affects more than 20 million Americans while rheumatoid arthritis affects more than 2 million Americans. Whereas rheumatoid arthritis affects 1 percent of the population, osteoarthritis affects virtually everyone as they age.

In osteoarthritis, the joint space narrows. There is friction and even loss of bone. Excessive weight can accelerate weight-bearing joint destruction, such as in the knee.

Rheumatoid arthritis results from the body's misdirected immune response which attacks the lining inside the joint (synovium). Rheumatoid patients complain of symptoms such as fatigue, weakness, low-grade fever and morning stiffness usually lasts more than an hour, food allergies, infections and leaky gut. Three times as many females develop rheumatoid as men. Emotional or physical stress typically worsens symptoms. [FDA Consumer, June 2000]

What is America going to do with a hobbled population of adults who are still working, living longer, but disabled due to arthritis? More than 40 million Americans suffer with arthritis. More than half of arthritis sufferers experience some disability 10 years after diagnosis. The hip, knee and hand are the primary joints affected.

FAILURE OF MODERN TREATMENT

T. McAlindon, one of the leading researchers in collagen replacement for degenerative joint disease, wrote a letter in a major medical journal suggesting the use of glucosamine is the "dawn of a new era."

Non-steroidal anti-inflammatory drugs are the standard treatment for symptoms, but they may produce side effects (gastric ulcers, death) and may even worsen the osteoarthritic process. [Lancet 357: 251-56, 2001] In 1985 researchers reported on the use of non-steroidal anti-inflammatory drugs and destruction of the hip joint in osteoarthritis. The majority of the users of anti-inflammatory drugs (31 of 37 patients) experienced destruction of the hip joint. A much smaller percentage (12 of 33) experienced the same problem among the group that did not take anti-inflammatory drugs. Greater destruction of the acetabulum, the area at the head of the long-leg bone (femur) that comprises the top of the hip joint, was associated with use of anti-inflammatory drugs. The researchers said the bone destruction "gives cause for concern," since hip replacement surgery would be required which has a relatively high mortality rate in the

HA is the cushioning at the end of bones. Anti-inflammatory drugs relieve pain but produce greater wear and tear in the joint.

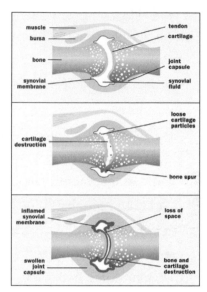

Photo: US FDA

elderly. [The Lancet 2: 11-14, 1985] The pain relievers don't restore the cushioning to the ends of bones. But the patient, feeling less or no pain, participates in more physical activity which in turn results in more wear and tear of the joints. It's obvious that pain relievers may dampen symptoms but accelerate joint destruction.

JOINT SPACE

A more comprehensive way of evaluating therapy for arthritis is to examine the effect of treatment upon the root cause of the problem --- bone rubbing on bone. Maintaining the space between the joints is critical. In one study it was shown that among patients who took 1500 milligrams of glucosamine sulfate for three years, there was no significant change in the narrowing of the joint space. This sounds disappointing till one examines the control group that did not supplement their diet with glucosamine and only took pain-relieving anti-inflammatory drugs. The non-glucosamine users experienced a significant narrowing of the joint space. While glucosamine only produced modest benefits in regards to symptoms, the deterioration of the joint had apparently been halted. Furthermore, there were no adverse reactions with glucosamine compared against non-steroidal anti-inflammatory drugs which can cause stomach ulcers and even death. [J COM, 8: 11-12, 2001]

The superiority of glucosamine sulfate and other natural pro-collagen supplements is seen in a study conducted in China. Among 178 patients suffering from osteoarthritis of the knee, one group received 1500 mg of glucosamine sulfate while the other was given a daily 1200 mg dose of ibuprofen. Both regimens reduced symptoms, but glucosamine sulfate was much better tolerated with 16 percent of the patients experiencing adverse reactions from ibuprofen compared to just 6 percent with glucosamine. Furthermore, 10 percent of the patients taking ibuprofen had to stop taking the drug whereas none of the glucosamine patients experienced side effects serious enough to stop their supplementation. [Arzneimittelforschung 48: 469-74, 1998]

ANTI-INFLAMMATORY DRUGS

Physicians admit that currently available drugs for arthritis are disappointing. [Clinical Journal Pain 17: 25-32, 2001] The fact that anti-inflammatory drugs reduce pain but slightly worsen joint deterioration has been known since 1985. [Lancet 2: 11-14, 1985] Go ahead, do like that television commercial shows and celebrate, celebrate! Take those new COX2 inhibitor arthritis drugs. You may be feeling less pain but your bones are paying a price.

Non-steroidal anti-inflammatory drugs (NSAIDS) work by inhibiting an enzyme called COX2. Newer COX2 inhibitors reduce gastric ulcer problems but still do not eliminate the risk. These COX2 inhibitors don't block the enzymes (TNF-alpha and IL-1B) that destroy cartilage. For comparison, a natural herbal extract from nettle leaf (urtica dioica) reduces TNF-alpha and would be more beneficial. [FEBS Letters 442: 89-94, 1999]

Another serious problem with common anti-inflammatory drugs is that they can eat a hole in your digestive tract which can result in bleeding. Some of these cases are uncontrollable and an estimated 16,5000 people die and over a hundred thousand are hospitalized annually in the USA. Most of these people are arthritics who die needlessly from a bleeding ulcer caused by use of a pain reliever. [Postgraduate medicine 109: 117-28, 2001]

About half of the American population is infected with H. pylori, the germ that causes stomach cancer and gastric ulcers. H. pylori infection may aggravate the toxicity of NSAIDS, and thus, H. pylori and ulcers should be treated prior to the use of these drugs. [J Gastroenterological Hepatology 15: G58-68, 2000] But which doctor attempts to kill off the H. pylori before prescribing the non-steroidal drugs? VIOXX (refecoxib) and Celebrex (celecoxib) were approved in 1998-99 to treat arthritis. Both drugs lower the relative risk of stomach ulceration, however both drugs still carry a warning label that they can cause ulcers, mortal ulcers.

Aspirin and the non-steroidal anti-inflammatory drugs work by inhibiting production of hormone-like substances called prostaglandins. But there are beneficial and harmful prostaglandins and these pain relieving drugs do not distinguish between them. So the prostaglandins that repair cartilage are also inhibited. This is a likely reason for the accelerated destruction of the joints with the use of these drugs. [Am J Medicine

81-36, 1986; Lancet 2: 519, 1989] Aspirin increases the risk of bleeding anywhere in the body and retinal hemorrhages have been linked with chronic aspirin use.

Tylenol (acetaminophen) is a potent pain reliever but it is toxic to the liver and accounts for 70,000 plus annual visits to hospital emergency rooms for liver toxicity and is responsible for a number of deaths and liver transplant operations annually. Kidney failure is another problem with acetaminophen-based pain relievers. People who consume a Tylenol capsule every day have twice the risk of losing their kidneys compared to those who take less can 104 capsules per in a year. [New England Journal Medicine 331: 1675, 1994] Recently VIOXX, the popular painkiller, has been linked to cases of nonbacterial meningitis and this should be added to the list of side effects for this drug. [Associated Press, March 25, 2002] There are 52 million Vioxx prescriptions written annually.

IRON IN THE JOINTS

The lack of HA would mean bone is rubbing on bone. The particular free radical that breaks down HA is the superoxide radical, the same radical that jolts iron free from circulating blood cells called phagocytes. Various iron binding metal chelators can effectively prevent the degradation of HA, but not EDTA a common chelator

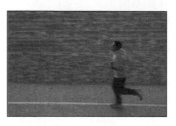

Morning is a good time for physical exercise. Patients with rheumatoid arthritis experience morning stiffness due to the overnight pooling of hyaluronic acid in the joint.

often used by alternative medical doctors. Iron and/or high amounts of vitamin C may be able to depolymerize HA. During inflammatory diseases the iron content of synovial fluid sharply rises. Iron in synovial fluid rises by a factor of six times in rheumatoid arthritis. Free iron plus vitamin C accelerates the degradation of HA. [Journal Inorganic Biochemistry 14: 127-34, 1981] Of all the agents that can degrade HA, free iron is by far the most powerful. [Carbohydrate Research 22: 43-51, 1972]

SYNOVIAL FLUID AND HA

Joint (synovial fluid) has a tiny amount of HA, approximately 0.15 percent hyaluronic acid. [Carbohydrate Research 32: 228-34, 1999] Yet HA plays such an important role in maintaining joint health. Normal synovial joint fluid contains 3-4 milligrams per milliliter of HA at a molecular weight of 4-5 million

Daltons. In osteoarthritis HA levels in synovial joint fluid drops to 1-2 milligrams per milliliter and 1-4 million molecular weight.

In the 1970s injection of HA into the knees of lame race horses was successful in returning these animals to the race track. [J Am Veterinary Assoc 58: 1132-40, 1997]

The first studies of HA in the treatment of osteoarthritis in humans were conducted in the early 1970s in South Africa, the USA and Britain using HA of 2-3 million molecular weight. [Pathological Biology 22: 731-36, 1974] In 1987 two commercial low-molecular weight (500,000-700,000) HA products (Artzal and Hyalgan) were administered by injection and were shown to reduce pain, improve function and produced results equivalent to non-steroidal anti-inflammatory drugs. [New Frontiers in Medical Science: Redefining Hyaluronan, Elsevier Science, 2000, p. 89-103]

HA, MORNING STIFFNESS AND EXERCISE

The level of HA in blood serum increases with physical exercise. Activity forces the broken down HA out of the tissues and into the blood plasma and lymphatic system. In the early morning the blood plasma levels of HA are low and the excess HA in the joints puffs up the joint with water which results in morning stiffness in cases of arthritis. The fluid in the joint is too viscous. Within a half hour to two hours after rising in the morning the blood serum concentrations of HA rise with the activity levels of the patient. Muscular activity pumps the excess HA out of the joints via the lymphatic system into the general circulation and morning stiffness subsides. [Scandinavian Journal Clinical Lab Investigation 48: 765-70, 1988; The Biology of Hyaluronan, CIBA Foundation Symposium 143, John Wiley & Sons, 1989, p. 233-47] So the best time to take HA supplements for adults with morning stiffness is midday, when the excess HA has had a chance to get pumped out of the joints. Therefore the morning is a good time to exercise.

GLUCOSAMINE SULFATE

Glucosamine sulfate is a starting block for the production of HA. Glucosamine is a widely used drug in Europe but is a food supplement in the USA. It is a naturally occurring substance produced by cells called chondrocytes. Glucosamine appears to stimulate the chondrocytes to produce the water-binding HA and chondroitin sulfate and it inhibits certain enzymes which destroy cartilage.

In a review of studies using nutritional supplements for arthritis, of 13 studies reviewed for glucosamine sulfate,

13 were positive; of 4 studies using chondroitin sulfate, all 4 were positive compared to taking a placebo pill. Discrepancies in studies may be indicative of variable product quality offered in an array of brands at health food stores. [Rheumatic Disease Clinic North Am 25: 379-95, 1999] Another review of 15 studies where glucosamine sulfate was employed in joint disease, a modest improvement was noted overall with some studies showing major beneficial effects. [J Am Medical Assn. 283: 1469-75, 2000] Glucosamine is essentially only half of the HA molecule, yet it produces positive results.

CHONDROITIN SULFATE

In degenerative joint disease there is a loss of chondroitin sulfate. Chondroitin sulfate is a major component of cartilage. It is a large molecule comprised of many linked molecules of glucosamine sulfate. CS helps to preserve chondrocytes (cartilage cells) from death. [Presse Medicale 27: 1859-61, 1998] Chondroitin stimulates production of cartilage and retains water for lubrication in the joint.

Only about 10 to 15 percent of chondroitin is absorbed orally while about 90+ percent of glucosamine is absorbed. An oral dose of chondroitin sulfate has been shown to increase blood plasma levels of CS which is evidence that it is successfully absorbed. [Arzneimittelforschung 45: 918-35, 1995] Low molecular weight CS is more readily absorbed. About 13 percent of CS of low molecular weight (5000 Daltons) has been shown to be absorbed in one study. [Arzneimittelforschung 41: 768-72, 1991] Other studies confirm that 10 to 20 percent of low-molecular weight CS (5000 Daltons) is orally absorbed. [Int Journal Pharmacological Research 13: 27-34S, 1993] Orally administered CS (800 mg per day) elevates levels of CS measured in the joint synovial fluid and was found to be superior to indomethacin and ibuprofen anti-inflammatory agents. [Osteoarthritis Cartilage 6: 14-21S, 1998]

CS oral supplementation (1200 mg/day) for several months has been shown to reduce the need for anti-inflammatory drugs among arthritic patients by 67 percent (nearly half of cases of arthritis needed no anti-inflammatory drugs at all!). [Presse Medicale 27: 1866-68, 1998]

Researchers have determined that 800 mg of CS taken daily reduces the time it takes to walk 20 meters. [Osteoarthritis Cartilage 6: 31-36A, 1998] Functional impairment of patients with osteoarthritis of the knee is reduced by approximately 50 percent after a year of taking 800 mg of CS. [Presse Medicale 27: 1862-65, 1998]

Six-month supplementation with 800 mg of chondroitin sulfate reduced joint pain in patients with osteoarthritis of the knee. [Osteoarthritis Cartilage, May 1998]

McAlindon's review of studies using glucosamine and/or chondroitin showed that chondroitin was superior to glucosamine. [J Am Med Assoc 283: 1483-84, 2000]

COMBINED GLUCOSAMINE AND CHONDROITIN

In 1999 reviews of studies using glucosamine and chondroitin began to be published. Of six studies using glucosamine and seven using chondroitin, there was a statistically significant improvement overall in all 13 studies, though it was modest, when these agents were compared to taking placebo tablets. In one study, glucosamine was superior to ibuprofen and another study it was equivalent. Most of these studies dealt with pain relief and improvement in mobility, not actual improvement in the bone-on-bone condition that causes osteoarthritis. [Rheumatologic Disease Clinics North America 25: 379-95, 1999]

HA INJECTIONS

HA injections aren't new. In 1988 in Italy arthritic patients received HA injections and improvement in joint mobility, pain, and reduced analgesic consumption were noted. [Clinical Therapy 10; 521-26, 1988]

There is a great deal of controversy over the effectiveness of HA injections in joint disease. David T. Felson MD of the Department of Medicine at the Boston Medical Center, writes that HA is cleared from the fluid compartment of the knee after only a few hours. The commercial HA products used for injection are designed to remain within the joint longer. But only modest increases in HA levels in the knee joint, about 10 percent, have been measured 2 to 22 days following injection. In horses, the increase in HA in the knee joint only lasted for two days. While Dr. Felson uncovers evidence that NSAIDS are far more effective than HA injections, he is comparing apples to oranges. The drugs only mask the symptoms while HA restores the joint. Larger studies appear to show little or no benefit from HA injections, Dr. Felson claims. [Archives Internal Medicine 162: 245-47, Feb. 11, 2002] However, HA and chondroitin appear to halve the degeneration of the joint. Pain relievers don't do this. With all of the controversy, researchers have concluded that hyaluronic acid "represents a substantive addition to the therapeutic armamentarium in osteoarthritis." [Current Rheumatology Reports 2: 466-71, 2000]

The concentration and molecular weight of HA determine the properties (viscosity and elasticity) of synovial fluid. In osteoarthritis the HA is both smaller in size and lower in concentration. Injection of HA of various molecular weights has been shown to be effective. Products are medium molecular weight Orthovisc, Synvisc (cross-linked high molecular weight), and low-molecular weight Hyalgan and ARTZ. [Drug Safety 23: 115-30, 2000] However, the benefit of HA in the synovial joint fluid is not always related to its viscosity, concentration or molecular weight. Researchers believe there may be some other pharmacological property in HA, rather than a physical property, which is beneficial in joint disease. [Journal Rheumatology 21; 297-301, 1994]

ORAL HA, CHONDROITIN SULFATE

Dr. K. Morrison of Fresno, California reports an unpublished study providing oral doses of Bio Cell Collagen II, which provides 50 milligrams of HA per capsule in a base of Type II collagen and chondroitin sulfate. Four capsules per day were taken prior to meals by 89 individuals who experienced pain from osteoarthritis, gouty arthritis, rheumatoid arthritis, post surgical and post traumatic pain, lumbosacral and cervical spine pain. Some of the patients received the Bio Cell Collagen II and others received a placebo, and then the two groups switched medications. Within 45 days 89.9 percent of the subjects taking BioCell Collagen II reported subjective relief from pain, most within 21 days.

ONE PHYSICIAN'S REPORT ON THE USE OF BIOCELL COLLAGEN II FOR 45 DAYS AMONG 89 PATIENTS WITH VARIOUS FORMS OF ARTHRITIS.

DAYS TO RESPONSE	0 - 7 DAYS	8 - 2 1 DAYS	21-45 DAYS	TOTALS
RHEUMATOID ARTHRITIS	9	6	3	18
OSTEOARTHRITIS	7	12	5	24
FIBROSIS	4	7	2	13
LUMBOSACRAL/ HERNIATED DISC	3	6	6	12
POST TRAUMA PAIN	2	4	3	9
GOUTY ARTHRITIS	2			2
CERVICAL SPINE/ HERNIATED		1	1	2
PLACEBO			(1)	(1)
REPORT PAIN RELIEF				80
NO PAIN RELIEF				9
TOTALS	27	36	26	89

Side effects: one patient reported nausea (also nauseated with other medications). Most subjects had been on long-term medication therapy.

RHEUMATOID ARTHRITIS

Rheumatoid arthritis is a completely different and less common form of arthritis. It usually begins earlier in life, around age 40, and is more common in females as are all autoimmune diseases.

In rheumatoid arthritis the body's immune system is attacking the joint. The degradation of HA is accomplished via attack by oxygen radicals, the rusting agents of the body. Iron chelators completely protect HA from this assault while SOD and catalase, other antioxidants produced naturally within the body, offer only partial protection. [Journal Rheumatology 22: 400-05, 1995] But natural iron chelators (bioflavonoids, IP6 rice bran extract) for unexplained reasons are largely unused in the treatment of rheumatoid arthritis.

Blood serum HA levels have been found to be higher among rheumatoid arthritis patients compared to osteoarthritis patients. [Clin Chim Acta 181: 317-23, 1989] This probably means more HA is being degraded by the autoimmune attack on the joint. Low-molecular weight HA is produced in the joint fluid of patients with rheumatoid arthritis, whereas high-molecular weight HA is produced in healthy tissues. This means the HA is really being chewed up.

Injection of HA into the knee joint of patients with rheumatoid arthritis has been shown to improve symptoms. [Clinical Experimental Rheumatology 19: 377-83, 2001]

As a percentage of the US adult population, the incidence of rheumatoid arthritis shrunk between 1985-1994 from 61.2 to 32.7 per 100,000 population. [Arthritis Rheumatism 46: 625-31, 2002] This is probably due to the aging of the population. Rheumatoid arthritis affects adults beginning around age 40 or so. Osteoarthritis, the wear-and-tear type of joint disease, begins around age 60. As more Americans live longer there will be a dramatic shift in the percentage of rheumatoid arthritis cases to osteoarthritis cases.

ORAL TOLERANCE

Rheumatoid arthritis is a disease where the immune system deciphers joint collagen as being "foreign" and attacks it like it were attacking a tumor cell or a germ. There has been an effort to de-sensitize this undesirable autoimmune reaction by providing very small amounts of native, undenatured collagen in oral doses. Oral tolerance is an approach to suppress the autoimmune reaction by stimulating the natural mucosal immune mechanisms in the gut associated lymphoid tissues of the small intestine. To suppress the autoimmune reaction, oral delivery of an appropriate amount of protein may slowly dampen the undesirable response. For arthritis, the protein that is used is Type II collagen. These proteins are broken down into fragments by digestive processes. Small doses of these proteins then begin to induce the oral tolerance effect. [Immunology Today 18: 335-43, 1997] This approach to treatment of rheumatoid arthritis appears to have some merit.

In one study, 0.25 milligrams (just 1/4th of a milligram) a day of oral Type II chicken collagen was employed among 60 rheumatoid arthritis patients to produce oral tolerance. While two patients experienced remission from the disease, statistically Type II collagen was ineffective. [Clinical Experimental Rheumatology 18: 571-77, 2000]

Type II collagen has been administered in doses of 20, 80 and 320 micrograms in mice. The lowest dose aggravated the disease but the highest dose induced tolerance by suppressing the immune response. [Arthritis Rheumatism 44: 1917-27, 2001]

In 1993 Harvard researchers reported that the use of Type II collagen among 60 patients with rheumatoid arthritis decreased the number of swollen and tender joints over a 3-month period but not in those who received an inactive placebo tablet. Four patients experienced complete remission from the disease. The patients were given 0.1 to 0.5 milligrams of Type II collagen orally. [Science, Sept 24, 1993] Administration of Type II collagen by oral or nasal administration in mice produced suppression of TNF-alpha and Interleukin-6 in the joints. [Journal Autoimmunity 13: 315-24, 1999]

Some companies that market oral collagen supplements are causing a great deal of confusion among patients with arthritis. Oral tolerance is an approach exclusively for the treatment of rheumatoid arthritis which affects less than 5 percent of the population. [Baillieres Clinical Rheumatology 10: 41-54, 1996] Yet companies keep marketing their oral native chicken collagen products, claiming they are superior to other denatured (hydrolyzed) collagen products which are designed for use among patients with osteo arthritis. Native chicken collagen has only been demonstrated to be effective when taken in very small doses, and only among rheumatoid arthritis sufferers. See the section near the end of this book which helps consumers understand the health claims of these products.

HA AND THE KNEE JOINT

About six percent of the adult US population age 30 years and older suffers from osteoarthritis of the knees. While anti-inflammatory drugs and exercise have been shown to be helpful in relieving symptoms, total replacement with an artificial knee implant is the sole remaining treatment when all other efforts fail.

Examination of the knee joints of dogs reveals the areas which exhibited osteoarthritis were the knee compartments that displayed a significant loss of HA. The molecular weight of the HA in dogs with osteoarthritic changes has not been shown to differ from that of normal healthy dogs. [Arthritis Rheumatism 31: 538-44, 1988]

Females experience more knee injury and arthritis than males. One reason for this may be that estrogen alters collagen synthesis in the knee ligaments. Type I collagen increases as estrogen levels rise. Progesterone has a dampening effect on estrogen's Type I collagen production. [Clinical Orthopedics 383: 268-81, 2001] Another reason is that women's hips are wider and the leg bones come down at an angle to the knee, resulting in different forces on the female knee joint than males.

The injection of HA has been shown to be effective in relieving pain among patients with osteoarthritis of the knee. [Clinical Orthopedics 385: 130-43, 2001] There is little question that HA injections in the knee reduce symptoms of pain and inflammation. However, 3 to 5 injections are generally required to achieve results. [Nederlands T Genees 144: 2188-92, 2000]

Among 108 patients with osteoarthritis of the knees, five weekly injections of HA produced relief from symptoms as early as 4 weeks after treatment in 68 percent of patients. [American Journal Orthopedics, Supplement, Nov. 1999]

HA may also be good for knee ligament tears. In an animal study, the knee ligaments (anterior cruciate) were lacerated on both sides and then healing was observed. In 14 of 21 rabbits treated with HA, their healing was superior to that of animals that just had salt solution injected into their joints. There was less inflammation in the HA-treated rabbit knees. [J Orthopedic Research 8: 425-34, 1990]

HA AND THE SHOULDER

Patients with "frozen shoulder" benefit from HA injections. [Int Journal Tissue Reaction 20: 125-30, 1998]

HA AND THE HIP JOINT

It has been reported that hip dysplasia in breeds of dogs depends upon their HA levels. The Australian Kelpie has a low incidence of hip dysplasia and a relatively high concentration of HA in joints compared

Some patients with capral tunnel syndrome report remission of symptoms after taking oral hyaluronic acid.

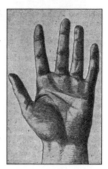

to Alsatians who commonly experience hip problems. [Medical Hypotheses 23: 171-85, 1987]

HA AND CARPAL TUNNEL

Patients with carpal tunnel or shoulder pain exhibit four to five times greater concentration of HA in their blood serum than healthy individuals. [Artificial Organs 18: 420-24, 1994] This indicates loss of HA from the joint.

HA AND TMJ JOINT

Complaints of painful arthritic joints and Temporal Mandibular Joint jaw pain often are common companion symptoms. [Cranio 16: 230-35, 1998]

In an experiment the TM joints in animals were intentionally roughened and then the animals were split into two groups with one group receiving HA injections. The group of animals receiving the HA had fewer degenerative changes. [Journal Veterinary Medical Science 63: 1083-89, 2001]

Chondroitin sulfate also appears to be an important type of collagen that prevents temporomandibular joint pain. [Journal Oral Maxillofacial Surgery 56: 199-204, 1998]

HA injections have been shown to be effective in reducing TMJ joint problems. [Journal Craniomaxillofacial Surgery 29: 89-93, 2001] HA injections in cases of TMJ often results in relief of symptoms and a greater range of movement. [Int Journal Oral Maxillofacial Surgery 30: 194-98, 2001]

In a study of patients with TMJ, oral glucosamine sulfate (500 mg/day) was compared to ibuprofen, an anti-inflammatory drug. Improvement was noted by 71 percent of the patients taking glucosamine sulfate and 61 percent of the patients taking the pain reliever. Glucosamine sulfate increased daily function and continued to provide relief after supplementation was stopped. [Journal Rheumatology 28: 1347-55, 2001]

HA AND DISCS

One study found no significant differences in HA or chondroitin sulfate in the intervertebral discs of normal and symptomatic adults. [Clinical Orthopedics 293; 372-77, 1993] In fact, in acute cases of disc herniation, more HA is found. [Z Orthop Ihre Grenzgeb 137: 211-13, 1999] This is possibly an indicator of a healing process.

HA AND SACROILIAC JOINT

HA has been injected into the sacroiliac joint with successful results. [Regional Anesthesia Pain Medicine 24: 84-88, 1999]

METAL CHELATORS AND JOINTS

In 1982 the journal Arthritis and Rheumatism reported that metal chelators inhibit the breakdown of HA. [Arthritis Rheumatism 25: 1469-76, 1982] Yet today, two decades later, the use of metal chelators to treatment arthritis is largely ignored.

The physiological concentration of HA in healthy joint fluid ranges from 2.50 to 3.65 milligrams per milliliter. Iron induced free radicals readily degrades HA. [Annals Rheumatic Disease 50: 389-92, 1991] HA break down is facilitated by ascorbic acid in the presence of free iron and free iron or copper in the presence of oxygen, which causes HA to lose its viscosity. Since synovial joint fluid has little natural antioxidant protection (superoxide dismutase or catalase activity), it is likely protected from degradation by natural binders of iron and copper, such as ceruloplasmin, transferrin and albumin, which are produced in the liver. [Journal Inorganic Chemistry 34: 69-74, 1985]

Laboratory studies indicate oxygen radicals do not depolymerize HA but rather alter its molecular configuration. Only when iron is added to the HA is the molecular weight diminished. [Annals Rheumatic Diseases 50: 389-92, 1991]

To maintain HA, adults should consume more fruits, grapes, berries, tea and other herbals as well as whole grains that contain the metal chelator IP6. Food supplements that provide these natural iron binders are readily available.

HA AND CHONDROITIN SULFATE VS ANTI-INFLAMMATORY DRUGS

Chondroitin sulfate and HA appear to have superior qualities over anti-inflammatory drugs.

First, chondroitin sulfate has been compared to anti-inflammatory drugs in the treatment of arthritis. Italian researchers tested chondroitin sulfate and diclofenac (Voltaren), an anti-inflammatory drug, among 146 patients with osteoarthritis of the knee. Patients either took 1200 mg of chondroitin or 150 mg of the drug. Patients taking the drug experienced pain relief but these pains reoccurred when the drug was stopped. Whereas when chondroitin was stopped, the pain relief lingered for up to three months. [Journal Rheumatology 23: 1385-91, 1996] So long-lasting relief is produced by chondroitin sulfate.

Another study showed that HA was as effective as medical therapy (Naproxyn) over a 26-week period but the patients were required to undergo five weekly HA injections. [J Rheumatology 25: 2203-12, 1998]

Second, chondroitin sulfate is less troublesome. A study compared the provision of 1500 milligrams of glucosamine sulfate to 1200 milligrams of ibuprofen among patients with osteoarthritis of the knee. Both medications significantly reduced symptoms of knee pain and swelling but glucosamine was better tolerated than ibuprofen. Only 6 percent of the glucosamine group versus 16 percent of the ibuprofen group reported side effects and none of the patients who took glucosamine had to drop out of the study compared to 10 percent among the patients who took ibuprofen. [Arzneimittelforschung 48: 469-74, 1998]

Third, HA appears to be equivalent to steroids in the treatment of arthritis [Drugs 47: 536-66 1994] without all of the side effects produced by steroids (poor wound healing, cataracts, glaucoma, many others).

COMBINATION NATURAL JOINT THERAPY

One researcher has suggested an extensive regimen of food supplements that would include niacinamide, glucosamine, SAMe, fish oil and selenium in the treatment of osteoarthritis. [Medical Hypotheses 53: 350-60, 1999]

CHAPTER SEVEN

HA and the Eyes

The eyes are one of the organs with very high concentrations of HA. HA plays a major role in maintaining the health of the ocular tissues such as the cornea (clear front window of the eyes), the retina, the vitreous gel that fills most of the eye, and the drain (trabecular meshwork) that maintains fluid pressure inside the eye. The high HA content of the human eye may explain why the provision of oral HA supplements has been reported to have profound effects upon vision in some people.

All of the factors that can break down HA can come into play in the human eye. Since the human eye is transparent to light, solar ultraviolet radiation can attack the cornea on the surface of the eyes as well as the inner eye structures such as the lens, vitreous gel and retina. Riboflavin, vitamin C and potentially toxic metals such as iron and copper are all found in eye tissues. In a test tube, German scientists grew retinal tissue and exposed it to high levels of riboflavin, iron and ultraviolet radiation. The combination inhibited the growth of retinal nerve cells. [Free Radical Biology Medicine 24: 798-808, 1998]

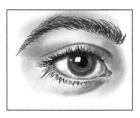 **The eyes are one of the organs with very high concentrations of HA.**

HA AND THE FLUID DRAIN (GLAUCOMA)

The common form of glaucoma has been called an HA deficiency. [Medical Hypotheses 51: 483-84, 1998] Glaucoma, which affects the eyes of about 2 percent of the total population, but as much as 8 percent of aged adults, is characterized by poor outflow of aqueous fluid from the inner portion of the front of the eye which then builds up pressure and may pinch off the branch-like network of optic nerves at the back of the eyes. This can result in narrowed side vision. Conventional treatment of glaucoma with medications, that reduce the flow of aqueous fluid, can effectively reduce intraocular pressure but may induce cataracts and other side effects. So a preventive measure would be welcome.

The link between a shortage of HA and glaucoma is compelling. Aqueous fluid drains out of the eyes through a mesh-type filter composed of collagen. There is less HA in the fluid drain of aging eyes. [Z Gerontol 23: 133-35, 1990]

In 1996 researchers examined the eyes of recently deceased aged individuals. The normal fluid drain of the eye (trabecular meshwork) of individuals who had glaucoma had 77 percent less hyaluronic acid than normal eyes. Six of ten eyes examined had no detectable HA whatsoever. [Investigative Ophthalmology 37: 1360-67, 1996] This is compelling evidence that a shortage of HA in the human eye is linked with age-related eye disorders.

The aqueous fluid of adult eyes may contain five times more HA than the fluid obtained from children. [Current Eye Research 16: 1069-71, 1997] This probably means that more HA is being lost with advancing age and is being washed from the eyes.

The cells in the fluid drain of the eyes produces less HA among glaucoma patients. The addition of vitamin C to these cells stimulates the production of HA. [Z Gerontol 26: 243-46, 1993]

Vitamin C may be an antidote to this problem. Aqueous fluid is normally high in vitamin C. When additional vitamin C is added to aqueous fluid in a laboratory dish, HA production is elevated. [Z Gerontology 26: 243-46, 1993]

In hypothyroidism the abnormal accumulation of HA residue in the fluid drain of the eye may result in poor outflow and elevated fluid pressure. A rise in eye fluid pressure has been reported in a hypothyroid patient who discontinued thyroid hormone medication. [J Am Optometric Assoc 67: 109-14, 1996]

It is known that steroids can raise the fluid pressure in the eye. It has been shown that steroids impair the production of HA in eye tissues. [Experimental Eye Research 64: 539-43, 1997]

Eye surgeons have successfully placed a net-like HA implant into the eyes of patients with advanced forms of glaucoma. This HA implant is a very hopeful new anti-glaucoma therapy. [Journal Cataract Refractive Surgery 25: 332-29, 1999]

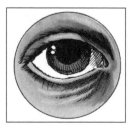

The common form of glaucoma is believed to be caused by a deficiency of hyaluronic acid.

HA AND THE OPTIC NERVE

Chondroitin sulfate is the major support collagen for the optic nerve. [Investigative Ophthalmology 35: 838-45, 1994] Research studies show that HA is virtually absent from the insulation (myelin sheath) that surrounds certain types of optic nerve bundles among patients with glaucoma (open-angle). Decreased amounts of HA may make the nerves prone to damage from elevated fluid pressure in the eye. [Experimental Eye Research 64: 587-95, 1997]

HA AND THE VITREOUS GEL OF THE EYE

The vitreous jelly of the eye is almost completely water (97%) with some collagens and HA. The makeup of healthy vitreous collagen is 92 percent HA and 8 percent chondroitin sulfate. [Biochemistry International 25: 397-407, 1991]

With advancing age the vitreous jelly of the eye begins to lose its consistency, the HA releases water and clumps of HA as well as watery patches appear much like a bowl of Jello looks after it has been stored in the refrigerator for some time. [Albrecht Von Graefes Klin Exp Ophthalmology 196: 187-97, 1975]

This HA breakdown can result in what are called floaters, clumps of protein in the vitreous body that interfere with light traveling through the eye. Floaters appear as cobwebs or insects floating in or in front of the eye.

What causes the breakdown of HA? Because of the transparency of the human eye to light, the vitreous jelly is prone to breakdown by solar ultraviolet rays. Iron, copper, excessive riboflavin or viral attack are other factors that break down HA in the eye. [Current Eye Research 13: 505-12, 1994] When vitreous jelly obtained from animals is exposed to light from a fluorescent lamp along with the administration of riboflavin, the jelly liquefies. Free, unbound copper or iron also induces this destructive process. The addition of vitamin C along with these metals further increases the liquefaction. [Nippon Ganka Gakkai Zasshi 99: 1342-60, 1995]

With advancing years, the vitreous jelly can also shrink and detach from its contact with the retina (called a posterior vitreous detachment), an event that is often accompanied by showers of floaters and what appear to be sparks of light in the field of vision. The injection of the enzyme that degrades HA, hyaluronidase, into the vitreous of animal eyes has been shown to induce a posterior vitreous detachment. [Retina 18: 16-22, 1998] Antioxidant enzymes like superoxide dismutase or catalase, which are produced naturally within the body, and iron chelators may be helpful in preventing or reversing some of the aging changes observed in the vitreous. [Intl Journal Biological Macromol 22: 17-22, 1998] There is more HA in the vitreous of normal eyes compared to ones where the vitreous has detached. [Graefes Arch Clin Exp Ophthalmology 223: 92-95, 1985]

In a laboratory test, iron chelators inhibited the breakdown of HA obtained from the vitreous gel. Diabetics experience accelerated breakdown of the vitreous due to HA decomposition. [Internatl Journal Biological Macromolecules 22; 17-22, 1998] Diabetics are prone to develop breakdown of the vitreous jelly of the eye due to the degradation of HA. Iron chelators prevent this from occurring. [Internatl Journal Biological Macromolecules 22: 17-22, 1998]

As the vitreous gel degrades and liquefies it becomes watery and thus no longer pushes up against the retina to keep it in place. Retinal detachments are also more likely to occur, particularly among people who are highly nearsighted or diabetics. The breakdown of HA in the vitreous in diabetic retinopathy and retinal detachment have been exclusively associated with the breakdown of HA. [Albrecht Von Graefes Klin Exp Ophthalmology 196: 187-97, 1975]

HA has been found to be a safe vitreous substitute. [Ophthalmic Research 29: 409-20, 1997]

To protect against the age-related breakdown of the vitreous body inside the eyes, protective UV-blocking

Degraded hyaluronic acid makes the eye prone to floaters and retinal detachments.

sun lenses should be worn during daylight hours spent outdoors. Excessive riboflavin (more than 10 milligrams) should be avoided in food supplements. High-dose vitamin C is not harmful unless there is iron overload in the vitreous body. Buffered vitamin C powder usually is accompanied by bioflavonoids which are iron binders, and thus this is the ideal form of vitamin C.

HA AND CATARACTS

In the human eye the aqueous fluid bathes the inner eye and delivers vitamin C, glutathione and other antioxidants that help reduce inflammation and retain the clarity of the focusing lens of the eye. However, if vitamin C levels in the lens drop significantly, this permits riboflavin to become oxidized by solar ultraviolet radiation which could result in discoloration of the lens, loss of transparency and a cataract. [Photochemistry Photobiology 72: 815-20, 2000]

High amounts of hyaluronic acid (HA) are found in the vitreous jelly of the eye. Unfiltered sunlight, excessive riboflavin, infections and inflammation may degrade HA in the human eye.

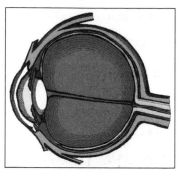

HA AND THE RETINA

The loss of HA production at the back of the eye with advancing age may play a role in the onset of retinal disorders. [Archives Ophthalmology 111: 963-67, 1993] Researchers have discovered that the retina and its blood supply layer (choroid) of the human eye exhibits no HA after the fifth decade of life.

HA is a component of the material between the millions of light-receptor cells in the human retina. [Journal Cell Science 114: 199-205, 2001] Collagen helps to support the light receptor cells (called rod and cones) and its primary component is HA. HA is damaged when retinal detachments occur. [Hyaluronon organization of the interphotoreceptor matrix of the retina, J.G. Hollyfield, www.glycoforum.com]

Among patients with age-related retinal (macular) degeneration, the sclera or white of the eyes becomes rigid, which indicates of loss of HA. [Ophthalmology 96: 104-08, 1996

In the white sclera of the eyes the loss of moisture increases with age by about 1 percent per decade. [Mechanics Ageing Development 77: 97-107, 1994]

HA may be of therapeutic benefit to patients with Stickler's syndrome, an inherited disorder characterized by retinal detachments, joint problems, cataracts and facial and dental abnormalities. [Acta Ophthalmologica 59: 286-95, 1981]

Excessive thyroid hormone (hyperthyroid) has been shown to reduce the production of HA in cells that guard the retina. [Ophthalmic Research 31: 399-406, 1999]

HA AND THE CORNEA

The abnormal deposition of HA in the healing cornea may reduce corneal transparency. [Investigative Ophthalmology Visual Science 35: 2774-82, 1994]

Pterygia are abnormal pinkish growths that grow across the front of dry eyes. Pterygia are rich in HA. [Japanese Journal Ophthalmology 30: 165-73, 1986]

HA AND DRY EYES

The front surface of the eyes, the cornea, is bathed in tear fluid that is secreted from water, oil and mucin-secreting glands in the eyelids. A shortage of these tear-film components may result in symptoms of redness, itching or burning of the eyes, or what is called dry eyes. The conventional treatment is to use artificial tears.

HA eye drops have been shown to be superior to some other types of eye drops in relieving dry eye symptoms among users of computer terminals. [Experimental Eye Research 68: 663-39, 1999] HA eye drops have been proven effective in reducing damage to the cornea caused by dry eyes. [British Journal Ophthalmology 86: 181-84, 2002] Both chondroitin sulfate and HA eye drops have been shown to relieve symptoms of dry eyes. [Am Journal Ophthalmology 103: 194-97, 1987]

HA may be a more effective agent in encouraging healing in the cornea than antibiotics. Researchers suggest non-infectious cases of corneal erosion could be treated with HA eye drops. [Eye 12: 829-33, 1998]

HA is an excellent lubricant for contact lens wearers. [Contact Lens Association Journal 21: 261-64, 1995]

The use of an HA solution on the eyes during laser-assisted corneal re-shaping surgery improves the surgical results in all cases studied. The corneal surface was smoother. [Ophthalmology 108: 1246-60, 2001]

CHAPTER EIGHT

HA and Cancer

HA presents one of the most promising approaches to cancer therapy and prevention.

HA has a dual nature in regards to cancer. [European Journal Cancer 37: 849-56, 2001]

Intact HA can keep tumor cells planted at their site of origin, preventing them from growing and spreading, while broken down HA can facilitate invasion and spread of tumors (metastasis).

The gold standard in cancer therapy is survival, not shrinkage of tumor size or reduction in the number of tumors. Conventional therapy is highly inflammatory, toxic and lethal. Thus most cancer patients succumb to treatment rather than the disease.

Survival is dependent upon keeping the initial tumor locked in the closet so to speak. If it doesn't spread (metastasize) it's not likely to be mortal. Tumors can grow and cause pain by pressing on nerves, but they have great difficulty doing any further damage by themselves.

Hyaluronic acid has a dual nature in cancer.

To spread, tumor cells must first create some space around them to move. Since the connective tissue fills in space around cells, movement of abnormal cells is inhibited. It's kind of like a tumor cell's feet being planted in hardened cement. The HA and connective tissue serves as a barrier for the spread of tumors.

Cells adhere to each other. The cells that can easily move and break away are found in the epithelia, the surface layers, of the skin, stomach, lungs, mouth and other organs. The majority of tumors begin in epithelial tissue. In cancer cells the adhesion molecules that keep cells together are partly or entirely missing. Degraded hyaluronic acid binds to the surface of a tumor cell and gives the cell "roller skates." HA can facilitate slippery movement of the tumor cells. In order to spread (metastasize), tumor cells must be able to avoid adhesion (sticking) to other cells, detach from the tumor mass and pass through barriers in the connective tissue. The connective tissue is largely composed of hyaluronic acid and chondroitin sulfate.

Tumor cells can break down this barrier via enzymes, such as hyaluronidase and also metalloproteinase. [Int J Cancer, March 12, 2002] Hyaluronidase is the same enzyme found in snake and insect venom which causes toxins to spread. Hyaluronidase is produced in tumors such as melanoma, colon carcinoma and certain brain tumors.

If the HA breaks down due to exposure to radiation, either x-ray, gamma ray or solar radiation, or due to viral or bacterial infection, or inflammation, then the connective tissue loses its consistency and any existing tumors cells can use the slipperiness of the watery HA to travel to distant locations. For example, the recurrence rate for colon cancer after an operation increases from 20 to 80 percent as the levels of HA increase in cancer cells. [Cancer Research 58: 342-47, 1998

Once detached, a cancer cell can make its way into the blood or lymphatic circulation. This is why surgeons often remove the lymph glands surrounding an excised tumor. Once in the lymphatic system the prognosis for cure drops significantly.

Hyaluronidase also enables tumor cells to avoid adhesion, make their way through the connective tissue barriers to release growth factors that promote the development of new blood vessels. The new blood vessels are then used as a conduit to provide nutrients for tumor cells to grow.

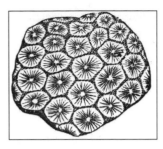

Hyaluronic acid (HA) holds malignant cells in place. Once HA is broken down, tumor cells can migrate, a grave condition which is called metastasis.

The native, high-molecular weight HA can only form into small fragments that facilitate the growth and spread of tumors if the HA is broken down by enzymes such as hyaluronidase and metalloproteinases. This is why hyaluronidase blockers such as iron-binders (bioflavonoids, phytic acid IP6) are so important. High-dose vitamin C can also play a preventive role by inhibiting the production of hyaluronidase which helps to "wall off" tumors. [Alternative Medicine Review 3: 174-86, 1998]

New blood vessels also create an exit for tumors cells to leave their site of origin. Once in the blood circulation, the cancer cells try to reattach themselves elsewhere. Very few, maybe 1 in 10,000 cancer cells survive the circulatory system where they are exposed to an array of immune soldiers such as macrophages, T cells, natural killer cells and other immune factors. The tumor cell may not even travel far, becoming trapped in the first set of capillaries downstream from the mother tumor, which is often in the lungs or the liver, which are frequent sites of metastasis.

HA: BARRIER AGAINST CANCER

In 1986 O.J. Stone proposed that HA and the entire matrix of connective tissue is an important barrier against the growth and spread of tumors. Stone wrote that anything that helps to retain the viscosity (consistency) of HA increases the body's resistance to tumors whereas enzymes like hyaluronidase, stimulated by infection or radiation exposure, encourage tumors. [Medical Hypotheses 20: 117-24, 1986]

The research work of Mary Helen Barcellos-Hoff at the Life Sciences Division, Lawrence Berkeley Laboratory, in Berkeley, California, helps to reveal the anti-cancer properties of HA and connective tissue in general. Ionizing radiation (x-rays) is a known cancer promoter, particularly in breast tissue. The radiation damages the matrix of material that surrounds cells, the HA and collagens. In an animal experiment, connective tissue that surrounds mammary-gland epithelial cells was exposed to low-dose ionizing radiation. Then non-irradiated breast gland cells were implanted within this matrix of connective tissue. A massive increase in tumors was observed in the non-irradiated mammary cells! More tumors occurred and arose more quickly and grew larger compared to non-irradiated animals. Only 19 percent of non-irradiated connective tissue produced small, infrequent tumors versus 81 percent tumor incidence (larger more frequent tumors) in irradiated connective tissue! The tumors grew so fast in the mammary cells implanted in irradiated connective tissue that by 6 weeks all of the mammary glands had tumors! Whereas only 39 percent of the mammary gland cells implanted in non-irradiated connective tissue expressed small tumors and some of these regressed and disappeared. The study had to be halted because all of the irradiated mammary gland cells were tumorous by the sixth week. Had the study continued, the difference between the two groups would have been greater because of the tumor regression observed in the non-irradiated animals.

Previously the connective tissue was believed to be an uninvolved bystander to cancer. It is now obvious that disrupted connective tissue permits the initial tumor cells to proliferate. As Barcellos-Hoff says, "Indeed, it has been suggested that cancer may be a physiological response to an abnormal environment." Studies reveal there are many more mutated cells produced that can initiate cancer than actual number of tumors that develop. The initiation of cancer appears to be a far more frequent event than the cases of cancer that develop. Low-dose radiation upsets the environment surrounding cells

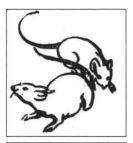 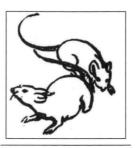

Irradiated mice   Unirradiated mice

Breast cancer cells placed in unirradiated connective tissue remain small and die off over time. Breast cancer cells placed in connective tissue exposed to radiation grow in number and size. Radiation may break down connective tissue (hyaluronic acid), which results in the spread of tumors. This calls into question the use of radiation to treat cancer.

and promotes tumors, an effect that lasts for 14 days following radiation exposure. By re-establishing the matrix of supporting tissue, tumors and pre-tumorous cell processes can be reversed, even in the presence of grossly abnormal genetically-damaged cells! [Cancer Research 60: 1254-60, 2000]

Barcellos-Hoff notes that conventional thought is the ionizing radiation promotes cancer by its ability to damage DNA. But her experiments clearly show that cells undamaged by radiation, but existing in an environment of connective tissue that has been irradiated, will aggressively grow tumors of large size and numbers. Barcellos-Hoff suggests it is possible to develop blocking agents to interrupt tumor progression. [Journal Mammary Gland Biology Neoplasia 3: 165-75, 1998]

Even more evidence of HA's anti-cancer barrier effect comes from Japan. Researchers at Osaka Medical Center for Cancer and Cardiovascular Disease report that removal of an extended zone of connective tissue in addition to lymph glands surrounding pancreatic tumors increased the 5-year survival rate from 8 to 25 percent. [Gan To Kagaku Ryoho 29: 364-69, 2002] This is an astounding improvement in survival for a type of cancer that traditionally has a very high mortality rate.

SHARK CARTILAGE DISAPPOINTING

The observation that tumors do not grow in cartilaginous tissues led to the idea that shark cartilage taken orally may serve as a treatment for cancer. While shark cartilage added to the diet of animals has been shown to delay the growth of tumors, it does not abolish their progression. [Anticancer Research 21: 10565-69, 2001] Cartilage is tissue that does not contain any blood vessels, and thus it is low in iron content. Cartilage inhibits the formation of new blood vessels which are required for tumor growth. But shark cartilage has not been proven in clinical trials to be of much benefit. [Biol Pharm Bulletin 24: 1097-101, 2001]

HA INTERCEPTS CANCER CELLS

Another intriguing quality of HA is that it has the ability to intercept roaming cancer cells. Cancer cells that metastasize (spread) make their way from the original tumor site through newly-formed blood vessels into the blood circulation. These roaming tumor cells have cellular parking spaces for HA. Dr. David C. Baker, Professor of Organic Chemistry at the University of Tennessee, has conducted research on short, low-molecular weight HA that immediately halts metastasis in mice. Short-length HA might attract migrating cancer cells and thus render them harmless. Think of an elaborate anti-missile defense system whereby incoming missiles (tumor cells) are immediately intercepted by HA before they can develop into a ball of tumor cells at a site distant from their origin.

While degraded HA at the site of a tumor may enable tumor cells to travel to distant locations, short-length, low-molecular weight HA introduced into the circulatory system may completely block the spread of cancer. Inhibition of cancer at 90-100 percent was achieved in animals with HA measured at 8-26 oligomers (dual strands) in length. No toxicity was observed. [Data: David C. Baker, U of Tennessee]

HYALURONIDASE AND CANCER

Hyaluronidase has been described as one of the "molecular saboteurs" to destroy HA. [Proceedings Natl Academy Sciences 93: 7832-37, 1996] The growth and spread of tumors is totally dependent upon new blood vessel formation. The process all starts with hyaluronidase, the body's own venom, inducing new blood vessel formation in tumor cells. Hyaluronidase inhibitors can block angiogenesis. [Proceedings National Academy Science 93; 7832-37, 1996]

In prostate tumors there is a high level of the HA breakdown enzyme (hyaluronidase). High-grade tumors have up to 20 times more of this enzyme than low-grade tumors. [Cancer Research 56: 651-57, 1996]

The Gleason (invasion) score is higher among prostate cancer patients who exhibit high hyaluronidase levels. Invasion of a prostate tumor outside the prostate gland was found in 83 percent of cases whereas no invasion was found among specimens where tumors remained local. [Oncology Reports 6: 1431-33, 1999]

Elevated levels of hyaluronidase correlate with invasive breast cancer. [Oncology Reports 6: 607-09, 1999] Invasiveness of breast cancer is directly related to elevated levels of hyaluronidase. Breast tumors exhibited four times more hyaluronidase than healthy breast tissue in one study. [Oncology Reports 6: 607-09, 1999]

Certain hyaluronidase inhibitors completely block hyaluronidase and angiogenesis (new blood vessel formation). A report in the Proceedings of the National Academy of Sciences says "a number of hyaluronidase inhibitors are readily available." [Proceedings National Academy Sciences 93: 7832-37, 1996] For example, a very low dose of green tea bioflavonoids provided in drinking water has been shown to prevent the growth and spread of colon cancer in rodents. [Japanese Journal Cancer Research 84: 1007-09, 1993] A patient with early-stage lung cancer has been reported to be successfully treated with an inhibitor of hyaluronidase. [Japanese Journal Clinical Oncology 7: 85-92, 1977].

New blood vessel formation is enhanced by fragments of HA and various growth factors, while intact HA, genestein from soy, heparin, cyclosporine A, and steroids are among an array of angiogenic inhibitors. [Internal Review Cytology 159: 113-60, 1995]

USING HYALURONIDASE TO TREAT CANCER

The dual nature of HA and hyaluronidase is sometimes perplexing. HA can help to keep tumors from spreading or it can promote the spread of cancer by the same process. (Remember, tumor cells borrow HA and use it as their "molecular roller skates" to travel to distant locations.)

The dual nature of HA and its breakdown enzyme, hyaluronidase, in cancer control needs to be recognized. A recent report said: "Paradoxically, both hyaluronic acid and hyaluronidase are involved in malignant transformation and cancer progression." Their mechanisms of action are not fully understood. HYAL-1 is the predominant form of hyaluronidase and the loss of HYAL-1 often correlates with tumor progression, particularly tobacco-related cancers. [Cancer Letters 163: 95-101, 2001]

Hyaluronidase can be employed in the treatment of cancer. HA hydrates, that is holds water, and thus over-production of HA can expand and open up spaces around cancer cells so they can find a pathway to invade surrounding tissues. Hyaluronidase is an enzyme that breaks down the HA and eliminates this mechanism. In studies where human breast cancer cells have been implanted in animals, hyaluronidase given intravenously shrinks the tumors to half their size in just four days. [Robert Stern MD, Univ. Calif. San Francisco] In Austria, doctors have used hyaluronidase to treat children with brain tumors and have produced favorable results. [Cancer Letters 131: 101-08, 1998]

Hyaluronidase is being successfully used to break down HA so that anti-cancer drugs can penetrate into areas of the brain where tumors reside. Children with brain tumors who received hyaluronidase plus chemotherapy faired better and had fewer relapses. [Cancer Letters 131: 101-08, 1998] Hyaluronidase is only available as a drug, not a food supplement.

In mice where melanoma cells had been implanted, the pre-administration of hyaluronidase before injection of an anti-cancer drug (vinblastine) was shown to produce marked anti-tumor effects. Hyaluronidase helped the drug to spread to the tumor. Hyaluronidase by itself did not alter tumor growth or metastasis. [Journal Cancer Research Clinical Oncology 121: 193-202, 1995]

BREAST CANCER

A remarkable study using oral chondroitin sulfate in animals shows that breast tumors can be completely inhibited. Oral chondroitin sulfate has been shown to reduce the incidence and size of mammary tumors in virgin female mice.

INCIDENCE OF MAMMARY TUMORS AFTER 18 WEEKS OF FEEDING CHONDROITIN SULFATE IN ANIMALS	
PURIFIED DIET	35.0%
PURIFIED DIET + 0.5 PERCENT CHONDROITIN SULFATE	28.6%
PURIFIED DIET + 1.0 PERCENT CHONDROITIN SULFATE	11.4%
PURIFIED DIET + 2.5 PERCENT CHONDROITIN SULFATE	0.0%
MORRISON LM, SCHJEIDE OA, CORONARY HEART DISEASE AND THE MUCOPOLYSACCHARIDES (GLYCOSAMINOGLYCANS), CHARLES C THOMAS, SPRINGFIELD, ILL, 1974.	

Female hormones affect HA and collagen production in the mammary glands. In rodents, estrogen and progesterone administered together elevate levels of chondroitin sulfate, HA and herparin sulfate. Estrogen alone elevates HA, while progesterone only elevates concentrations of chondroitin sulfate. In animals whose ovaries have been removed, progesterone alone or in combination with estrogen decreases levels of HA. [Acta Physiol Scandinavia 168: 385-92, 2000]

Elevated blood serum levels of HA are not found among breast cancer patients. [Int J Cancer 52: 873-76, 1992]

CANCER AND BLOOD LEVELS OF HA

Oncologists (cancer doctors) have been attempting to measure HA in the blood serum as a marker for tumors. However, HA is a poor marker for cancer because serum HA levels are not significantly elevated till the late stage of the disease. One would think as tumors destroy connective tissue that more HA would make its way into the blood circulation. But HA levels are not elevated in all types of tumors.

The concentration of HA in blood serum has not been found to be elevated in patients with sarcomas, lymphomas, brain tumors, breast carcinomas, and other malignancies, but is elevated by five-fold among patients with mesothelioma, a form of chest cancer, compared to healthy adults. [Cancer 62: 326-30, 1988] High HA serum levels have also been found in Wilms tumor. [Annals Medicine 28: 241-53, 1996]

SIZE OF HA AND CANCER

Landmark work conducted by Eva A. Turley and associates at the London Regional Cancer Center, University of Western Ontario, Canada, shows the size and concentration of HA determines HA's ability to inhibit tumors. Small fragments of HA may promote new blood vessel formation. These fragments are produced by hyaluronidase degradation of HA. [Cancer Letters 131: 21-27, 1998] High-molecular weight HA inhibits formation of new blood vessels while HA of a smaller size may stimulate the migration of tumor cells. [International Journal Cancer 60: 632-36, 1995] HA degradation which produces short-length HA, in the range of 2000-8000 Daltons or 4-25 disaccharides in length, stimulate the proliferation and migration of endothelial cells. [New Frontiers in Medical Sciences: Redefining Hyaluronan, Elsevier Science, 2000, pp. 77-86; Science 228: 1324-26, 1985] The small HA fragments are degradation products of HA. [CIBA Foundation Symposium 143: 187-201, 1989]

Please don't jump to the wrong conclusion here. Readers should not confuse the short, low-molecular weight HA generated naturally at the site of a tumor which facilitates tumor growth, with the short, low-molecular weight HA ingested orally or injected which can intercept roaming tumor cells. At the site of a ball of tumor cells short-length HA helps to spread cancer, whereas in the blood circulation it intercepts circulating tumor cells. Some researchers have become confused over this point and have mistakenly advised against the consumption of oral HA supplements for cancer patients.

BLOCKING THE CANCER RECEPTOR SITE

The Winnipeg Free Press in Canada reported a startling story of widespread interest on July 15th, 1995. The report said Manitoba scientists found they can stop the spread of cancer in mice by turning off a cancer cell's sensing ability. Sensors, called receptor sites, on the surface of living cells, are able to be knocked out and completely block the spread of a tumor. The knocked-out receptors later return to normal when the cancer risk has subsided. It's like pulling blinders over a cell. Tumor cells just die once they are blinded. [Winnipeg Free Press, July 15, 1995]

Millions of cancer cells are knit together in a ball, called a tumor. To spread the cancer, cells must be able to break free and travel to other sites. To do this the glue that keeps the cells together must weaken and the surrounding cement (connective tissue) must become mushy so the cancer cell can travel through it. Migrating tumor cells simultaneously emit paracrine growth factors that stimulate the host cell to produce hyaluronic acid. The metastasizing cell has a receptor (parking space) for HA which might attract cancer cells, but these cells are not attached to a tumor site and thus the circulating HA just takes them out of action. HA is an attractant for roaming cancer cells. Short forms of

Malignant cancer cells stick to hyaluronic acid.

HA are being developed to do this. The short-HA binds to tumor cells and prevents them from sticking to normal cells. Metastasis is halted.

HA and its cellular docking port (called a CD44 receptor) may promote the growth and spread of some but not all tumors. Strands (called oligomers) of 5-6 repeating dissacharides can inhibit tumor growth. HA is an ideal anti-cancer agent because it is naturally found throughout the body and is therefore nontoxic and is readily available to be harvested from animal tissues. [International Journal Cancer 77: 396-401, 1998]

For example, HA strands can be introduced into the body to bind to cell receptors (called CD44 and RHAMM) and compete with native HA. To determine whether this works, small osmotic pumps were used to slowly administer strands of HA to tumor sites in animals. As much as 80 percent inhibition of tumor growth was achieved. This was demonstrated over a period of 7-14 days with just 0.5 micrograms of the HA strand. [New Frontiers in Medical Sciences: Redefining Hyaluronan, Elsevier Science, 2000, pp. 51-62] See more on this below.

IRON, CHELATORS AND CANCER

Purified commercial HA contains significant amounts of iron. Additional iron causes HA to degrade. Ascorbic acid depolymerizes HA because it alters the form of iron (Fe^{3+} to Fe^{2+}). Iron chelators halt the degradation. [Journal Inorganic Biochemistry 14: 127-34, 1981]

In the presence of iron and hydrogen peroxide, D-glucuronic acid is converted into D-glucaric acid. [Carbohydrate Research 153: 119-31, 1986]

In a study conducted by the Center for Food Safety and Applied Nutrition at the Food & Drug Administration, phytic acid (IP6) was found to be a non-toxic metal chelator while other chelators were potentially toxic. [Environmental & Molecular Mutagenesis 38: 347-56, 2001]

GLUCURONIC ACID AND CANCER

The other half of the HA molecule is glucuronic acid. At the end of a woman's monthly menstrual cycle estrogen is dumped into the gut. Estrogen then couples up with glucuronic acid in the liver and then excreting it in the bile. Certain bacteria in the gut produce an enzyme, glucoronidase, which breaks the bond between estrogen and glucuronic acid, thus enabling estrogen to be reabsorbed back into the body. Calcium D-glucarate inhibits the glucoronidase enzyme, facilitating normal rather than elevated estrogen levels. In one animal study, two groups of rodents were studied. The rodents were bred to develop breast cancer. The animals were split into two groups and one group received calcium D-glucarate. Only 56 percent of the animals in the treated group developed breast tumors compared to 100 percent in the untreated group. Among the animals that did develop breast tumors, there were fewer tumors than normal. The number of tumors was reduced by 90 percent. The recommended consumption of calcium D-glucarate is 200-400 milligrams per day and more for individuals with existing breast cancer. [Israeli Journal Medical Science 31; 101-05, 1995]

High urinary levels of hyaluronic acid may be a marker for certain types of cancer.

BLADDER TUMORS AND HA

HA is involved in bladder cancer. High levels of HA (up 2.5-6.5 fold) and hyaluronidase (3 to 7 fold increase) are found in the urine of bladder cancer patients. Measuring the levels of HA and hyaluronidase in urine may help to diagnose bladder cancer. [Journal Urology 163: 348-56, 2000; Urologe 40: 121-26, 2001]

Hyaluronidase levels are 5-7 fold higher among patients with medium to high grade bladder cancer compared to healthy individuals. [Cancer Letters 131: 21-27, 1998]

Urinary levels of HA and hyaluronidase may indicate the presence of a bladder tumor. [Miami Nature Biotechnology Short Reports, The Scientific World 106SR, 2001]

In Canada, Bioniche Life Science, Inc. has been licensed to use Cystistat (hyaluronic acid) in Europe for the treatment of radiation cystitis, cystitis caused by infection or trauma, and neoplasia (cancer). Cystistat is injected directly into the bladder where it helps to restore tissues. [Doctor's Guide, Sept. 7, 2000]

PROSTATE CANCER AND HA

Three to eight times more HA is found in prostate cancer cells. [Journal Biological Chemistry 276: 11922-32, 2001] Prostate cancer cells often migrate to bone marrow. Increased HA levels apparently enhance the adhesion of prostate tumor cells to bone. [Journal Biological Chemistry 276: 17949-57, 2001]

SKIN CANCER AND HA

HA in the skin may last only a day whereas in cartilage it lasts for many days.

Hyal Pharmaceutical Corporation has received a patent for its Solarase product which combines HA and anti-inflammatory agents for the treatment of actinic keratosis, sun damaged skin. [Doctor's Guide, Jan. 21, 1997]

HA, DRUG COMBO

HA can be combined with anti-cancer drugs to target cancer cells. When HA is injected into rats who have liver cancer the HA targets and adheres to the cancer cells. Pre-treatment with chondroitin sulfate enhances the targeting effect. This means that HA could be used to selectively deliver certain drugs to cancer cells. [Glyconconj Journal 15: 935-39, 1998] There is an adhesion molecule that creates an affinity between cancer cells and HA. HA is an interceptor of cancer cells that are on the move. Pharmaceutical researchers have successfully combined HA with an anti-cancer drug (Taxol). This helps the drug in targeting the cancer cells. [Biomarcomolecules 1: 208-18, 2000] Other methods of targeting cancer cells, such as monoclonal antibodies, have failed because they only target the outside of the cancer cell but do not enter and destroy it. Because cancer cells utilize the cell receptors for HA in order to spread, the use of HA with an anti-cancer drug can help target the tumor cells better than use of the drug alone. [Pharmaceutical Research, Volume 19, April 2002]

SUMMARY

In summary, the best strategy to prevent cancer involving HA is to block its degradation. This keeps the cells that have turned cancerous in their place and keeps them from growing and spreading. It also hinders the development of new blood vessels (angiogenesis) that then feeds tumors nutrients required for their growth.

Natural iron chelators such as bioflavonoids (extracts from grape seed, bilberry, cranberry, blueberry, cherry, milk thistle, ginkgo biloba, green tea, quercetin, rutin, and others) and IP6 rice bran extract, or Echinacea, may be consumed from foods and supplements, to inhibit the production of hyaluronidase, the enzyme that breaks down HA.

Once cancer has begun to grow and spread, short-length, low-molecular weight HA taken orally may help to intercept circulating tumors cells.

Use of hyaluronidase to treat cancer should remain under a doctor's supervision.

The primary contraindication for HA among cancer patients is the occurrence of lymphedema (leg swelling). Cancer treatments may encourage the onset of lymphedema. Since HA thickens lymph fluid, oral HA supplements may worsen lymphedema.

CHAPTER NINE

The A-to-Z of Hyaluronic Acid

Hyaluronic acid and the various tissues or disorders of the body

Hyaluronic acid may play a preventive or therapeutic role in many other diseases or tissues in the body. Here is an A to Z list.

ALLERGY

Chondroitin sulfate inhibits the release of mast cells which are the triggers in inflammatory allergic reactions. Chondroitin sulfate has been found to be a stronger inhibitor of mast cells stronger than cromolyn, the drug most often used to treat allergies. [British Journal Pharmacology 131: 1039-49, 2000]

BLADDER

Cystitis is a painful disorder of the bladder characterized by urgency, frequency, pain and night-time urination. It occurs more frequently in females. About 8-60 cases per 100,000 females have been reported. Stress, certain foods and monthly hormone levels may worsen symptoms and patients often experience accompanying health problems such as allergy, irritable bowel and migraines. [Expert Opinion Investigative Drugs 10: 521-46, 2001]

In animals where cystitis has been chemically induced, HA injections have brought about improvement in bladder capacity. [Journal Urology 166: 710-13, 2001] Interstitial cystitis is an inflammatory condition of the bladder of unknown origin. One of the treatments for this condition is Cystistat, which is HA. It is not approved for use in the USA yet, but is undergoing clinical trials. In a study of 25 patients with interstitial cystitis in Canada, 40 milligrams of HA was instilled into the bladder weekly for 4 weeks, then monthly. By the twelfth week 71 percent of patients reported complete or partial remission. [Urology 49: 111-13, 1997]

HA also is helping children who experience abnormal urinary flow. In cases of vesicoureteral reflux, some of the urine in the bladder flows back into the ureters from the kidneys rather than from kidneys to ureters to bladder. This commonly occurs in young children following a urinary infection and may disappear as the child gets older. In a study conducted in Sweden, hyaluronic acid was instilled into the bladder. Among the 228 children treated with HA, 221 experience positive improvement and better than 8 in 10 had no need for subsequent surgery. [Journal Urology 166: 1887-92, 2001]

HA, ARTERIES AND CHOLESTEROL

Human male arteries are much richer in HA when young, but as they age the HA content drops and the accumulation of fatty deposits (triglycerides) increases. [Stroke 16: 687-94, 1985]

In animals provided a high-fat diet, the arteries tend to accumulate cholesterol deposits and the HA content decreases. [Artery 9: 44-58, 1981]

In animal tests, there is an accumulation of HA and a decrease in chondroitin sulfate in blood vessels when fatty plaques are intentionally produced. [Lab Investigation 33: 136-40, 1975] Arterial plaques are reduced in size with chondroitin sulfate. [Angiology 24: 269-87, 1973; Morrison LM, Coronary Heart Disease and the Mucopolysaccharides, C Thomas, Springfield, Ill, 1974]

Smooth muscle from human aorta was grown in a lab dish and placed in a high-LDL cholesterol or high-HDL cholesterol environment. High LDL cholesterol, but not HDL cholesterol, markedly decreased the HA

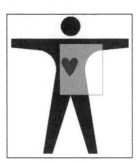

High levels of HA
improve the elasticity of
the aorta.

production. Cortisol, a stress hormone secreted by the adrenal glands, also inhibited the production of HA. [Artery 8: 323-38, 1980]

HA AND THE CAROTID ARTERY

In a study using rabbits fed a high-cholesterol diet, HA was administered shortly following an intentional injury to the carotid artery (neck artery). Usually following injury the macrophage cells accumulate at the site in such large numbers that they impair wound healing. But the provision of HA reduced the macrophage count and improved healing. [Atherosclerosis 114: 157-64, 1995]

HA AND THE AORTA

In animals it has been demonstrated that high levels of HA improve the elasticity of the aorta, the first major blood vessel outside of the heart. [Atherosclerosis 24: 259-66, 1976] High doses of vitamin C increase levels of HA and other forms of collagen in the aorta of rodents. [Atherosclerosis 19: 191-99, 1974]

In one study with diabetic rats, the HA content of healing aortic tissue increased by 44.7 percent, about the same as occurs in non-diabetic rats. But when the diabetic rats are treated with insulin the HA content of the aorta increases by 91.3 percent. [Journal Vascular Research 36: 209-21, 1999]

HA AND ANGIOPLASTY

Angioplasty has become popular since its introduction in 1979 for the treatment of arterial blockages. Instruments are inserted into the arteries to remove plaque and blockages. The initial success rate is around 95 percent but unfortunately blood vessels begin to narrow in 30-40 percent of cases within 6 months of the procedure. Researchers in France have found that HA cannot always bind to the arterial wall after these procedures, which is an underlying cause of angioplasty failure. By saturating HA into the arterial walls of animals who have undergone angioplasty, the HA can bind to the artery in place of the white blood cells (leukocytes) that usually interfere with the healing and rebuilding process. The researchers concluded that HA "may offer hope" in preventing the re-occurrence of narrowing in blood vessels following angioplasty. [Pathological Biology 46: 561-70, 1998]

Sometimes a stent or stainless steel support is implanted to prevent blood vessels from collapsing, but unfortunately the stent may attract blood platelets, which produces a clot. In lab experiments, HA coated stents inhibited the formation of clots. [Arteriosclerosis Thrombosis Vascular Biology 20: 1168-72, 2000]

HA AND BLOOD VESSEL GRAFTS

In rats, the provision of low-molecular weight HA prolonged the survival of grafted blood vessels. [Transplantation 69: 665-67, 2000]

HA AND HEART FAILURE

In rodents it has been shown that the amount of hyaluronic acid in cardiac tissues increases by three times within three days of an induced heart attack as the heart attempts to heal. The HA buildup then retains water which contributes to the swelling around the heart in heart failure. [Journal Clinical Investigation 88: 1622-28, 1991]

It has been shown that the amount of hyaluronic acid in cardiac tissues increases by three times within three days of an induced heart attack as the heart attempts to heal.

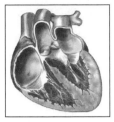

HA AND BLOOD PRESSURE

The drug lisinopril, an angiotension inhibitor, reduces fibrosis (scarring) in blood vessels of patients with high blood pressure. [Circulation 102: 1388, 2000] Patients with high blood pressure tend to have more collagen in blood samples. These patients may lack a chemical (hyaluronidase) that breaks down collagen. [Circulation 98: 535-40, 1998]

HA AND HEART FAILURE

Elevated blood levels of collagen may indicate heart failure. Lisinopril (Zestril, Prinivil) depletes the body of zinc and normalizes the collagen level. In rodents, the drug lisinopril has been shown to reverse stiffness of the heart tissues. [Hypertension 28: 269-75, 1996] Lisinopril has also been shown to inhibit cardiac scarring (fibrosis) in humans. [Circulation 102: 1388-93, 2000]

BLOOD

Both HA and chondroitin sulfate reduce the clotting time by 3-10 fold by binding with fibrinogen. [Biochemistry 26: 6052-57, 1987] High-molecular weight HA binds to fibrinogen, a clotting factor, better than low-molecular weight HA. [J Biological Chemistry 261: 12586-92, 1986]

Because HA decreases the clotting time of the blood by increasing the rate of fibrinogen production, HA could possibly be utilized to normalize clotting time among individuals with blood clotting disorders. [Cell Physiology 37: C952-57, 1995]

Abnormally high levels of HA may cause blood to become very viscous and coagulate (thicken and clot). This is observed in some cancer patients whose tumors cause tissue damage that releases more HA into the blood circulation. [American J Hematology 24: 247-57, 1987]

BRAIN

The loss of HA may explain why the brain shrinks over time. The average 50-year-old adult brain weighs about 3 pounds. Fifteen years later is weighs about 2.6 pounds. HA concentration in brain tissue decreases with advancing age. [CIBA Foundation Symposium 143: 208-20, 1989] HA plays the main structural role in the formation of the scaffolding that surrounds brain cells. [Anatomy Embryology 188: 419-33, 1993] The HA-rich environment of the brain is believed to be the reason why this tissue resists invasion by tumors originating outside the brain. [Glycobiology 6: 489-92, 1996]

Disease promotes loss of HA, which can be measured in cerebrospinal fluid.

DISEASE	RATE OF LOSS OF HA
HEALTHY ADULTS	166 MICROGRAMS PER LITER
BRAIN TUMOR	4000 MICROGRAMS PER LITER
MENINGITIS	8000 MICROGRAMS PER LITER
[ACTA NEUROLOGICA SCANDINAVIA 94: 194-206, 1996]	

HA is more abundant in young cerebral arteries than in aged ones. HA may play a role in stroke risk. [Stroke 16: 687-94, 1985]

DISC DISEASE

Discs that produce back pain have less HA and chondroitin sulfate and have less water content. [Clinical Orthopedics 293: 372-77, 1993] HA content in the disc rapidly decreases following herniation. [Spine 6: 194-210, 1981]

EARS

HA has been applied topically to the tympanic membrane in the ears to encourage healing of a perforated ear drum. [Acta Otolaryngology 110: 110-14, 1990]

In an animal study, HA-treated tympanic membranes of the ear closed faster and showed less scar tissue compared to natural healing. [Acta Otolaryngology 442: 54-61, 1987] Studies show that the use of HA during ear surgery protects the delicate hair cells. [Acta Otolaryngology 442: 62-65, 1987]

EPILEPSY

HA is believed to be involved in the transmission of nerve signals in the brain. HA may be involved in the transmission of GABA (gamma amino butyric acid). The inhibition of this neuro chemical may be involved in epileptic seizures. [The Biology of Hyaluronan, CIBA Foundation Symposium 143, John Wiley & Sons, 1989, p. 208-231]

ESOPHAGITIS

The main type of collagen in the esophagus is HA. The incidence of esophageal reflux (heartburn) in cases of collagen disease is about 10 percent. In scleroderma patients the incidence is about 50 percent. [Nippon Rinsho 58: 1908-10, 2000]

FIBROMYALGIA

Blood serum levels of HA are about 2.5 times greater in women with rheumatoid arthritis and nearly 10 times higher in women with fibromyalgia compared to healthy women. High circulating HA levels may be a diagnostic tool for these conditions. [Journal Rheumatology 24: 2221-24, 1997] Though there are contrary studies which show no increased HA levels in the blood serum of fibromyalgia patients. [Journal Rheumatology, 27: 2658-59, 2000]

GALLSTONES

Gallstones, particularly small ones, have very high levels of HA. High levels of HA in bile may play a role in the development of gallstones. [European Journal Hepatology 7: 135-40, 1995]

GRAVE'S DISEASE

In thyroid eye disease (Grave's disease), there are abnormal deposits of collagen (HA, chondroitin sulfate) that may result in eye bulging and an outward turn of the eyes. [Thyroid 8: 429-32, 1998]

HEADACHE

Following the fortuitous observation that glucosamine supplementation for arthritis relieved migraine headaches, a small study was conducted which showed that glucosamine produced a substantial reduction in headache frequency or severity. [Medical Hypotheses 55: 195-98, 2000]

Other studies indicate high-dose riboflavin (400 milligrams vitamin B2) may be used to treat migraine headaches. [Cephalgia 14: 328-29, 1994; Neurology 50: 466-70, 1998] High-dose riboflavin may encourage the breakdown of HA.

It is possible, that either by strengthening or weakening the wall of blood vessels in and around the eyes and forehead with glucosamine or riboflavin, that the blood vessel spasm that typically produces migraine pain is checked.

HEART

Certainly an antidote for heart and blood vessel disease has been overlooked. Chondroitin sulfate, known and utilized in recent years in the treatment of arthritis, was studied in the late 1960 and early 1970s by Dr. Lester Morrison of the Loma Linda School of Medicine. An initial group of 120 patients who either had coronary artery disease or had experienced a heart attack, were studied. Among 36 of these patients who received 1500-10,000 milligrams of chondroitin sulfate for 4 years, there were 4 coronary incidents and only 3 suffered a fatal heart attack. After four years, 27 of the 60 patients who did not receive chondroitin sulfate experienced 36 adverse coronary incidents and there were 9 fatal heart attacks.

FOUR-YEAR FOLLOW-UP OF PATIENTS WITH CARDIOVASCULAR DISEASE	
NUMBER OF SUBJECTS WHO DID NOT TAKE SUPPLEMENTAL CHONDROITIN SULFATE	
60 PATIENTS	27 OF THESE PATIENTS EXPERIENCED ADVERSE CORONARY EVENTS (45%)
NUMBER OF SUBJECTS WHO RECEIVED 10,000 TO 1,500 MILLIGRAMS OF CHONDROITIN SULFATE	
36 PATIENTS	ONLY 4 ADVERSE CORONARY EVENTS (11%)

There was a 600 percent decreased risk for an adverse event in the group that supplemented with chondroitin sulfate! There is no drug or treatment that can brag of such an effect today, over 35 years later! At the time, Morrison estimated that the use of chondroitin sulfate could potentially reduce the rate of acute coronary events in the USA to one-sixth of their level. He estimated the 500,000 annual deaths due to heart attacks and strokes could be reduced to under 100,000! No toxic effects were noted. The molecular weight of the chondroitin sulfate used was 29,500. When this was reduced to 3000-8000 the anti-blood clotting, anti-plaque properties were removed despite the fact that this lower-molecular weight product could be better absorbed. [Angiology 22: 165-74, 1971; Journal American Geriatrics Society 17: 913-23, 1969]

In another study, chondroitin sulfate has been shown to reduce cardiac events by 60 percent and reduce the death rate by 15 percent among patients with blood vessel disease. [Journal Intl Medical Research 6: 217-26, 1978]

Morrison also demonstrated the effect of chondroitin sulfate on rats. He gave the animals unusually high doses of vitamin D, a fatty vitamin, which raised their cholesterol. He then administered chondroitin sulfate to a group of the rats and fatty deposits in the blood vessels were not observed. [Proceedings Experimental Biology Medicine 131: 719-22, 1969] In 1968 Morrison also showed that chondroitin sulfate was superior to heparin sulfate as a blood thinner. Chondroitin prevented blood clots without interfering with the blood platelet count or plasma fibrinogen levels. [Journal Atherosclerosis

Research 8: 319-27, 1968] **Chondroitin** Morrison also demonstrated **sulfate heals a** the use of chondroitin sulfate **damaged heart** on adult squirrel monkeys who typically develop **and blood** high levels of cholesterol **vessels.** plaque as they age, just like humans. When chondroitin sulfate was administered to these animals the cholesterol plaques were completely abolished! They were completely absent. [Experientia 28: 1410-11, 1972]

Also in an animal study, Morrison intentionally fed rats a diet high in cholesterol and unusually-high amounts of vitamin D, a fatty vitamin, and observed abnormalities in the aorta of 17 of 18 animals. When the rats were fed the same cholesterol-elevating nutrients along with chondroitin sulfate, the aortic abnormalities were completely prevented. [Atherosclerosis 16: 105-118, 1972]

Morrison notes that chondroitin sulfate was first used in 1955 and demonstrated anti-plaque qualities in animal tests conducted in Japan. [Medical Journal Skiyshu University 1: 23, 1955] So humanity has ignored this evidence for over a half century.

In vitamin E-deficient rodents, the production of HA, chondroitin sulfate and other collagens decreased. The anti-blood clotting properties of vitamin E may be explained by its ability to maintain or increase the production of dermatan sulfate and chondroitin sulfate, both which thin the blood. [Atherosclerosis 55: 115-23, 1985]

HEART VALVES (MITRAL VALVE)

Viruses can induce the accumulation of HA in the myocardium. [European Journal Clinical Investigation 23: 277-82, 1993] This can lead to swelling of the heart valves.

HERNIA

The strength of the collagen matrix is important in preventing a hernia (rupture or bulging of tissue). Breakdown enzymes such as metalloproteinase can degrade tissue which may result in the development of recurrent hernias. [World Journal Surgery 10: 239-45, 2002]

HIP DYSPLASIA

Hip dysplasia in animals is usually treated with anti-inflammatory drugs. Recent reports of relief from symptoms of hip dysplasia with the use of glucosamine sulfate warrants further investigation. Joint laxity often accompanies hip problems, which is a sign that there is a shortage of HA and other types of collagen. [Veterinary Clinics NA Small Animal Practice 22: 595-606, 1992]

In dogs, hip dysplasia appears to be a consequence of lower HA levels in the joints. Joint abnormalities in dogs appears to arise "as a consequence of a deficiency in the levels of HA in synovial fluids." [Medical Hypotheses 23: 171-85, 1987]

INFECTION

HA is a barrier to protect against infection rapidly spreading throughout the body. Though infectious agents such as viruses and bacteria can break down HA, the HA slows its spread. For example, Streptococcus pneumoniae is a bacterium that causes pneumonia, meningitis, sinusitis and middle ear infection in humans worldwide, especially newborns and children. High concentrations of vitamin C are known to inhibit the degradation of HA by the destructive enzyme (hyaluronate lyase) which is produced by Streptococcus pneumoniae. High concentrations of vitamin C offer natural resistance to bacterial invasion by virtue of its ability to protect HA barriers. [Journal Biological Chemistry 276: 15125-30, 2001]

HA stimulates neutrophil functions, a certain type of white blood cell. HA may reduce the number of bacterial infections in susceptible humans. To test this, HA was injected under the skin of 29 patients with chronic bronchitis. HA-treated patients exhibited fewer infections and needed fewer antibiotics. One report says: "HA is a new substance that can be used to stimulate host defense reactions and reduce the need for antibiotics." [Am J Respiratory Care Medicine 153: 312-16, 1996]

KIDNEY

In kidney disease, increased levels of HA in the blood serum are a marker of progression of the disease. [Am Journal Kidney Disease 34: 1083-88, 1999]

HA is an important component of kidney stones in their early stage of formation. [Journal Urology 133: 319-23, 1985] However, while HA may induce the beginnings of small urinary stones, the administration of commercially supplied HA in a test environment did not encourage the development of stones near as well as HA obtained from stone formers. The crystallization-promoting property of HA does not apply to all individuals. [J Am Society Nephrology 14: 397-403S, 1999] Calcium oxalate crystals adhere to the surface of kidney cells. Administration of collagen (glycosaminoglycans) reduces adherent crystals. [European Urology 28: 68-73, 1995]

Chondroitin sulfate reduces the risk of kidney stones by lowering oxalate levels. [Urology 50: 173-83, 1997]

In diabetes, the sugar levels may stimulate HA in the kidneys which can lead to tubular fibrosis (scarring). [Metabolism 50: 789-94, 2001]

LIVER

High blood serum levels of HA occur in liver disease, such as hepatitis. The rejection of liver transplants can be measured by circulating HA levels. [Ann Med 28: 241-53, 1996] Elevated serum levels of HA may be an indicator of more progressive liver disease. [Journal Viral Hepatitis 5: 187-92, 1998]

If HA levels could be used to determine the stage of liver disease it may reduce or eliminate the need for liver biopsies. A liver biopsy is often performed prior to initiation of antiviral drug therapy. However, patients with hepatitis C are often not eager to undergo a liver biopsy. Some 30-40 percent of patients undergoing liver biopsy experience pain, and there can be severe complications including death (rare). A significant number of patients indicate they would not have a biopsy performed if they had been aware of the pain. [Am J Gastroenterology 96: 3053-55, 2001] More than 4 million Americans are infected with the hepatitis C virus and 30,000 new cases are reported annually. Corgenix Medical Corporation has acquired technology from Japan to perform a blood serum test that would measure levels of HA and may avoid the need for some liver biopsies. [Corgenix Medical, June 25, 2001]

Low-molecular weight HA given intravenously to mice can protect against liver failure. [Hepatology 34: 535-47, 2001]

HA in the blood circulation is routed to the liver when liver endothelial cells metabolize HA, that is, digest it. Each liver cell can bind many HA molecules. However, chondroitin sulfate is also bound to liver cells and has a higher affinity (by three-fold) for liver endothelial cells than HA. So chondroitin sulfate administered together with HA may minimize the amount of HA that is metabolized by the liver and thus help maintain higher circulating HA levels. [Biochemistry Journal 234: 653-58, 1986]

Low-molecular weight HA has been found to protect against inflammatory liver disease. This may be an important breakthrough for patients with liver disease who are being treated with immunotoxic drugs. [Hepatology 34: 535-47, 2001; Journal Immunology 165: 7150-56, 2000]

LOU GEHRIG'S DISEASE

Abnormally elevated levels of hyaluronic acid are found in the skin and blood serum of patients with amyotrophic lateral sclerosis. [Amyotrophic Lateral Sclerosis Other Motor Neuron Disorders 1: 213-18, 2000]

LYMPHEDEMA AND HA

Lymphedema is a swelling in the legs that often occurs following cancer therapy. As cancer therapy kills off living tissues, HA is degraded, and it makes it way through the lymphatic drainage system into the blood circulation, then to the liver where it is digested and removed in bile. [Connective Tissue Research 15: 33-41, 1986] Patients with lymphedema have much higher HA levels in their lymph fluid than normal healthy individuals. [Lymphology 31: 173-79, 1998] HA supplements, either oral or injected, should not be utilized among patients with a history of lymphedema. Leg swelling with the use of HA should prompt immediate cessation of the HA supplement.

MARFAN SYNDROME

HA-producing cells (fibroblasts) from Marfan syndrome patients produce 3 to 10 times more HA than normal fibroblasts. [J Biological Chemistry 254: 12199-203, 1979]

NERVES

Fragments of HA can be used to induce new blood vessel formation (angiogenesis) which is necessary for nerve regeneration. An injectable nerve guide can be placed near a damaged peripheral nerve and HA can be instilled. Following administration of HA, sciatic nerves in rodents exhibit better nerve conduction, have more nerve bundles and re-insulate (re-myelinate) more readily. [Journal Neuroscience Research 40: 318-24, 1995]

Under experimental conditions, HA has been injected into rodents via a guide into the sciatic nerve. The nerves exhibited improved activity. [Microsurgery 18: 270-75, 1998]

Researchers have shown if HA is combined with injectable anesthetics, blockage of pain or sensation is prolonged. [Anesthesia Analgesia 80: 740-46, 1995]

PROGERIA

Progeria is a rare disease with striking features that resemble accelerated aging.

The word is derived from the Greek and means "prematurely old." About 1 in 8 million births are progeria babies. Progeria kids have aged-looking skin, stiffness of joints, hip dislocations, heart problems and blood vessel disease, baldness and cataracts.

People with progeria live on average to the age of 13 and by the time they are six years old they look like they are 70 years of age. Progeria patients suffer delayed growth, a build up of fats and cholesterol in the arteries, cardiovascular disease and other maladies. Progeria patients have recently been found to have lower levels of antioxidant enzymes catalase and glutathione peroxidase. [Biochem Biophys Res Comm 257: 163-67, 1999]

Abnormally high urinary levels of HA are found in patients with progeria and Werner's syndrome. [Biochem Med Metab Biol 36: 276-82, 1986. In fact, progeria kids excrete 17 times more HA in their urine than healthy individuals. [Mechanics Ageing Development 35: 39-46, 1986] For unknown reasons, these children are losing HA from their bodies at a very rapid pace.

Some progeria patients exhibit low insulin-like growth factor and low human growth factor. Growth hormone injections improve growth in progeria patients. [Am J Clin Nut 55: 1222-24S, 1992]

The Hutchinson-Gilford progeria syndrome is a rare condition of unknown origin that results in failure to thrive, hair loss, stiffening of joints and severe blood vessel disease. The main cause of death is cardiovascular disease and the median life span is 13 years. Nutritional therapy and supplemental growth hormone improves growth and weight gain. [Metabolism 46: 851-56, 1997]

SCLERODERMA

Scleroderma means hard skin. It is a disease of connective tissue that lies beneath the skin and in between internal organs. Scleroderma is often preceded by and almost always accompanied by Raynaud's phenomenon, a circulation disorder characterized by sensitivity to cold which constricts blood vessels. When a wound occurs, collagen production rises and then falls, whereas in scleroderma it continues to produce collagen in an unstoppable fashion.

In scleroderma there is a progressive buildup of fibrous tissue. There is thickening and tightness of the skin about the fingers. Hair growth and sweating stop as the hair follicles and sweat glands are destroyed. Intense itching may be experienced. Lung fibrosis may cause shortness of breath. See the section in this book on fibrosis.

Oral Type II collagen has been shown to improve diseases of the intestines among patients with sclerosis. Sclerosis patients with ileus and other disorders improved and patients were able to tolerate foods. [Nihon Rinsho Meneki Gakkai Kaishi 22: 93-99, 1999] In aging sclerotic duodenum, the proportion of HA and CS decrease in patients with sclerosis. [Digestion 56: 230-36, 1995]

SCOLIOSIS

Birds with scoliosis, abnormally curved backbone, produce lower than normal levels of HA, while the levels of hyaluronidase, the enzyme that degrades HA, is abnormally elevated. [Biochim Biophys Acta 1034: 318-25, 1990] In young chickens, shortages of copper, manganese and vitamin B6 may induce scoliosis. [J Nutrition 117: 189-93, 1987]

SURGICAL ADHESIONS

HA minimizes the occurrence of adhesions. [J Surg Res 100: 217-21, 2001; Pharmatherapeutica 5: 233-39, 1988]

Postoperative adhesions are fibrous attachments between tissues. Adhesions frequently occur following abdominal or gynecological surgery. From 67-93 percent of patients undergoing these types of surgical procedures may experience pain from postoperative adhesions. Women may experience infertility due to adhesions.

Up to nine out of ten animals where HA was used immediately following surgery, prior to surgical wound closure, were free of post-surgical adhesions, versus 15 percent of operated animals who did not receive the gel. [Journal Surgical Research 100: 217-21, 2001. In another animal experiment, HA has been shown to prevent adhesions in hernia incisions. [Archives Surgery 137: 278-82, 2002]

In late 2001 the Food & Drug Administration approved Intergel (Lifecore Biomedical), a hyaluronic acid gel for use among women undergoing certain gynecologic surgical procedures. While Intergel is administered to reduce scarring, the FDA reports rates of infection may rise with use of the gel. Post-surgical infection rates rose from 2.9 to 5.6 percent with the use of the gel. While there are other adhesion-preventing treatments, this is the first that is liquid. [Neergaard L, FDA Approves controversial gel, Associated Press, Nov. 20, 2001]

THROAT AND VOCAL CORDS

One of the accompanying signs of aging is a guttural, dry sounding voice. People who are old sound like they have an "old voice" on the telephone. It's no wonder, since HA plays an important role in the shape and hydration of the vocal cords. Females exhibit a different distribution of HA in their voice cords than males, which makes them more prone to voice box injury. [Laryngoscope 111: 907-11, 2001]

HA plays an important role in the mechanical properties of the vocal cords. Removal of HA decreases the stiffness of the vocal fold cover. [Otolaryngology Head Neck Surgery 124: 607-14, 2001]

HA injections have been successfully performed in animal experiments and may prove useful in humans with a hoarse voice. [New Frontiers in Medical Sciences: Redefining Hyaluronan, Elsevier Science, 2000, p. 353-59]

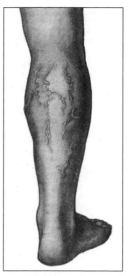

Varicose veins have lost collagen and accumulated hyaluronic acid. Herbs like grape seed extract and horse chestnut may be helpful in reducing varicose veins.

HA has been described as an ideal implant for scarred vocal cords. [Laryngoscope 109: 1142-49, 1999] Collagen injections in the vocal cords often produce satisfying results. [Am J Otolaryngol 14: 257-61, 1993]

One of the problems accompanying Parkinson's disease is speech abnormalities. Parkinson's patients often have a breathy quality to their voice, called hypophonia. It occurs as the tissues in the voice box stiffen. An injection of collagen (Zyplast) improved vocal qualities for two months in 11 of 18 patients treated. [Am Academy Otolaryngology, Sept. 10, 2001]

VARICOSE VEINS

More than 80 million Americans have a problem with the veins in their legs. One-way control valves in the leg veins help to push blood back towards the heart. When these valves don't work correctly, some blood may be allowed to flow backward and pool in the vein which stretches the tissue and causes a bulging known as varicose veins. More women than men experience vein varicosity. [J Am Academy Dermatology 46: 381-86, 2002] Aside from their unsightly appearance, symptoms include itching, swelling and aching legs. Treatment ranges from the use of surgical support stockings to vein stripping surgery.

Varicose veins have weak walls. Varicose veins exhibit high concentrations of water. [Israel Journal Med Science 33: 81-86, 1997] They have lost collagen and accumulated HA in the wrong spaces. Bioflavonoids are useful in protecting from the free-radical attack on veins. [Pathology Biology 43: 461-70, 1995] Fragments from veins of people with varicosity were grown in a laboratory dish. The addition of a bioflavonoid (grape seed extract) decreased the HA content by 34 percent. [Pathology Biology 45: 86-91, 1997]

An herbal product that is effective in the treatment of varicose veins is horse chestnut extract. Various studies indicate horse chestnut is as effective as surgical hose in reducing the fluid volume of the leg (-43.8 milliliters on horse chestnut versus +9.8 milliliters on placebo). Horse chestnut works by inhibiting the production of hyaluronidase that degrades hyaluronic acid. [The Lancet 347: 292-94, 1996; Archives Dermatology 134: 1356-60, 1998; BMC Cardiovascular Disorders 1: 5, 2001]

HA is also indicated in the treatment of deep vein thrombophlebitis. [Minerva Chir 33: 1581-96, 1978]

WOUND HEALING

HA is produced in wounded tissues. [Investigative Ophthalmology 35: 2774-82, 1994]

The model for perfect wound healing is the adult fetus. Wounds to a fetus heal with minimal or no scar formation. In the fetus, high levels of HA stimulate something called tumor necrosis factor alpha (TNF-A) which inhibits collagen production and thus limits fibrosis (scarring). [British Journal Plastic Surgery 50: 362-68, 1997]

In adults, HA levels are initially very low in fresh wounds and blood clots but increases as wound healing progresses. Clotting material (fibrinogen) and HA bind together, which facilitates the formation of a fibrin clot in the wound healing process. [J Theoretical Biology 119: 219-34, 1986]

The evidence that HA improves wound healing is overwhelming. For example:

HA slightly prolongs healing time but facilitates scarless wound healing. Healing in rodent skin was prolonged by two days (15.2 days compared to 13.4 days) when treated with HA versus a placebo, which inhibits collagen formation by promoting scarless wound healing. [Zhonghua Zheng Xing Wai Ke Za Zhi 16: 30-33, 2000] Among patients undergoing skin grafting following burn injuries, the application of HA to the burn wounds delayed wound healing by about a day. There was no evidence of less scarring. [Journal Burn Care Rehabilitation 17: 302-04, 1996]

The provision of an HA cream prior to radiation treatment helps to reduce swelling and wound healing. [Radiotherapy Oncology 42: 155-61, 1997] HA is transiently elevated in the granulation tissue during wound healing. [Wound Repair Regeneration 7: 79-89, 1999]

Skin wounds on diabetic rats heal better when HA is applied topically.
[J Surgical Research 35: 410-16, 1983]

The provision of HA in wound dressings is associated with brisker healing and reduced scarring. Oral glucosamine may be helpful following surgery or trauma to boost healing. [Medical Hypotheses 47: 273-75, 1996]

In Europe, HA used in a nasal cream following nasal surgery outperformed a conventional ointment in regards to healing time and prevention of crusting. [Drugs Experimental Clinical Research 25: 253-61, 1999]

HA skin grafts have been shown to be successful in healing diabetic foot ulcers. [New Frontiers in Medical Sciences: Redefining Hyaluronan, Elsevier Science, 2000, p. 313-20]

Adriamycin, an anti-cancer drug, may produce skin ulcers. The provision of hyaluronidase, the enzyme that breaks down HA, increases the ulcer rate by 50 percent in these chemotherapy patients. [Plastic Reconstructive Surg 101: 370-74, 1998]

In some wounds, the over-production of HA and collagen may induce scarring. Researchers are actually attempting to develop HA inhibitors that will minimize tissue fibrosis. [Biochim Biophys Acta 1495: 160-67, 2000] Researchers have demonstrated that L-arginine, an amino acid, inhibits the production of hyaluronan synthase, the enzyme required to produce HA. When L-arginine was administered to rabbits that had undergone surgical vein grafts, production of hyaluronan synthase was inhibited. Thus L-arginine could be employed post-surgically to prevent the re-narrowing of surgically implanted veins. [Journal Surgical Research 74: 39-42, 1998]

Even in healthy individuals, 500-3000 mg of vitamin C improves wound healing. [Oral Surg Oral Med Oral Pathology 53: 231-36, 1982]

WIDESPREAD MEDICAL APPLICATIONS

Additional medical applications of HA and its molecular cousin, chondroitin sulfate, are limitless. Here are a few.

Chondroitin sulfate sprayed into the nose reduces snoring. [Current Therapeutic Research 59: 234-43, 1998]

HA is a lubricating and healing agent in saliva so it may have therapeutic benefit among patients with dry mouth (Sjogrens' syndrome). [Archives Oral Biology 41: 667-71, 1996]

Cigarette smoke breaks down HA in the lungs of smokers. [Lung 167: 237-45, 1989] So oral HA supplements may be helpful in preventing various lung disorders associated with chronic tobacco use.

Chondroitin sulfate helps to prevent calcifications throughout the body and thus may be used as an alternative to calcium-blocking drugs. [Coronary Heart Disease and the Mucopolysaccharides, LM Morrison, CC Thomas, 1974]

Modern medicine's frustration in treating age-related joint disease may be overcome with a greater understanding of the role of HA in joint disease. Physicians frequently inject steroids (cortisone) into inflamed joints. Yet cortisone decreases HA levels. [Journal Investigative Dermatology 114: 953-59, 2000] So while inflammation subsides for awhile, the underlying root of the problem may be worsened by the use of anti-inflammatory drugs.

The link between stress and disease may be understood better with greater knowledge of HA. Cortisol, an adrenal stress hormone, decreases the synthesis of HA by 50 percent in a laboratory dish. [Atherosclerosis 35: 135-43, 1980]

Glucose and insulin reduce the amount of HA in cell dishes of human aortic smooth muscle cells. [European Journal Endocrinology 145: 193-98, 2001;

Arteriosclerosis Thrombosis Vascular Biology 20: 1480-87, 2000] Therefore, supplemental HA may be helpful for diabetics.

CHAPTER TEN

Commercially Available HA Products

For thousands of years medicine men ground up human and animal tissues for medicinal purposes. These ancient medicines are thought to be archaic if not bizarre by modern medicine. The Egyptian Ebers Papyrus, approximately 1550 BC, provides explicit instructions on how to prepare extracts of various organs including the liver, eyes and testes. Organs like the eyes, which are the richest natural source of hyaluronic acid and other collagens, are akin to the use of HA, chondroitin and glucosamine food supplements today.

Injectable HA products are many. Your physician will inform you of the appropriate types of injectable HA utilized in joints, skin, eye and other tissues. There is no sense in providing a list of all the available injectable HA products to consumers other than to note that some injectable HA products are derived from animals while others are synthetically produced. This may be an issue for people who wish to avoid animal products.

There is a growing list of available HA products for oral consumption. These products vary by their source (animal or synthetic), molecular weight, and dosage. It's important for consumers to recognize that the human body contains about 14,000 to 16,000 milligrams of total HA, and the body degrades and regenerates about 3000-5000 milligrams of HA a day. In an adult, particularly after age 60, there is about a net loss of 150 milligrams of HA per day. This loss of HA is believed to bring about many of the gradual aging changes observed in the human body. Provision of enough HA to produce a positive effect is important. Some oral HA products provide too little HA to produce any kind of positive effect.

Oral HA supplements certainly may have advantages over injectable HA since they do not require needles or physician office visits. Furthermore, once absorbed, oral HA would be available throughout all human tissues. Injectable HA is only available in the local area under treatment. For example, Restylane is a stabilized non-animal HA product of Swedish origin. It is provided in 0.7cc syringes for injection. It would take 200 of these injections to equal what the body normally loses in a day.

Ideally a good oral HA product should provide an adequate dose (more than 100 milligrams per day), be of low-molecular weight to facilitate oral absorption, and should be affordable. The accompaniment of other collagen sources, such as Type II collagen and chondroitin sulfate, which boosts HA levels on its own, is desirable. The extracellular matrix, often referred to as connective tissue, is composed of structural proteins (collagen and elastin), specialized proteins (bibrillin, fibronectin and laminin) and proteoglycans (sugar-like molecules). There are at least 12 types of collagen. Type II collagen is the common type found in cartilage and joints.

Additionally, the simultaneous provision or consumption of iron-binding antioxidants such as bioflavonoids and phytic acid IP6 rice bran extract, and vitamin C to aid in collagen formation, would be advantageous. Quercetin is a natural histamine blocker, which means it inhibits excessive acid formation in the digestive tract that can interfere with HA absorption and availability. The various oral HA products are presented below for reader review:

Biocell Collagen II™ (BioCell Technology LLC, Anaheim, Ca.) is a unique patented form of hyaluronic acid provided in a base of chondroitin sulfate and hydrolyzed Type II collagen. It is derived from young chick sternum collagen. Its molecular weight is 1500-3000 Daltons (low). It is provided in capsules providing 50 full milligrams of HA, 100 mg of chondroitin sulfate and 500 mg of Type II collagen. Consumers are instructed to take 3 capsules daily just prior to meals (before high stomach acid levels are achieved). For accelerated effect, consumers may wish to take 6 capsules a day for the first 45 days. Product analysis of BioCell Collagen II™ by Integrated Biomolecule Corp. verifies that this product is greater than 10 percent hyaluronic acid, 25 percent chondroitin sulfate. [Test, Lot No. 012322588, Feb. 21, 2002] Each lot of BioCell Collagen II™ is tested for HA content. Molecular weight was confirmed in the range of 800-2500 Daltons.

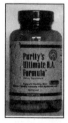 Purity Products in New York provides BioCell Collagen II™ in its Ultimate H.A. Formula in the above dosages along with quercetin as a stomach acid inhibitor, IP6 rice bran extract as a metal binding antioxidant and vitamin C.

Purity Products also offers a product called Vitalamax that provides the following ingredients. Hard Shell Gelatin Capsule: Each 2 capsules contain:

LETTER FROM A USER OF BIOCELL COLLAGEN II™

"In December 2001 I heard a radio broadcast about hyaluronic acid. In the program it was discussed that through a study of a Japanese farm culture a specific substance (HA) had been identified as most likely resulting in decreased signs of aging in that community. As a 52-year-old woman, I was intrigued with the skin and joint benefits, which were discussed as an attribute of this supplement.

I have taken the HA formula twice a day since receiving it in mid-December. I wanted to wait for about six weeks to see any results in the health of my skin. However, before that period of time was up, I began seeing improvements in my health, which I believe are directly related to this product.

Specifically, I had experienced increasing problems with hot flashes and night sweats. After four weeks of taking the HA supplement, I found I was experiencing milder and less frequent instances of hot flashes or night sweats. I continued from that time on to improve in these symptoms and now virtually do not have any problem.

I am prompted to write to recommend this product be investigated by others in my situation."

CL
March 27, 2002

VITALAMAX FROM PURITY PRODUCTS

HYALURONIC ACID (FROM BIO CELL COLLAGEN II 500 MG)	50 MG
ALPHA LIPOIC ACID	20 MG
BORAGE OIL	200 MG
FOLIC ACID	400 MCG
COD LIVER OIL (OMEGA 3)	300 MG
VITAMIN B12 (METHYLCOBALAMIN)	200 MCG
VITAMIN B6	10 MG
BETA CAROTENE (VITAMIN A ACTIVITY)	2500 IU
VITAMIN E (MIXED TOCOPHEROLS)	15 IU
FERULIC ACID (RICE BRAN)	35 MG
VITAMIN C (MAGNESIUM ASCORBATE)	60 MG
IP6 RICE BRAN EXTRACT	25 MG
CO-Q10	20 MG

A variety of BioCell Collagen II™ has been formulated for use with pet animals and grape seed extract, curcumin and pine bark extract added and is sold under the brand name ProMotion by Animal Health Options in Colorado.

Injuv™ is an HA food supplement provided in a soft gel capsule. Made by Soft Gel Technologies, Inc. it provides 6 milligrams of HA in 70 milligrams of an extract obtained from cockscomb. An enzyme cleavage technique is said to reduce the molecular weight of this product and facilitate oral absorption. Studies published by the manufacturer confirm that the product is absorbed orally. In animals, the addition of HA to the diet improved wound healing. In human studies, remarkable benefits were achieved in a short period of time. In just six weeks, taking 6 capsules providing 6 milligrams of HA per capsule (total 37.8 mg HA per day), for 45 days, among 96 women ages 22-65 years at Ohtsuma University, Japan, the following results were reported. About two thirds of the subjects reported improved smoothness in their skin and great flexibility in their joints and about a third surprisingly reported improvement in their eyesight. [Data: Soft Gel Technology]

Nu-Life by Kinetic Technologies provides 20 milligrams of synthetically-produced HA (molecular weight 500,000) in a capsule for oral consumption. Also offered are HA supplements for animals.

A widely advertised liquid HA formula, produced from natural sources, does not describe the origin of the material. It's manufacturer claims a few thousand patients have taken this product with beneficial results. The amount of HA in it is not provided in printed literature. Other sources indicate that this liquid formula provides 2.15 milligrams of HA per drop and the suggested dosage is 7 drops a day, taken orally. It is provided in a half-ounce bottle (217 drops). Claims have been made that this product is superior because of its high molecular weight (which should impair absorption), but cites as evidence a study where high-molecular weight HA was injected, not taken orally. [Clinical Therapeutics 20: 410-23, 1998]

Cyvex Nutrition markets a product Arthrocoll™, advertised as the purest Type II collagen of low molecular weight derived from the entire carcass of animals, but it does not provide HA or chondroitin sulfate. It does dissolve well as it is hydrolyzed.

Velvet antler, the renewed seasonal antler from elk approximately 60 days into its growth cycle which is covered with skin and a fine velvet-like layer of hair, is a rich source of nutrients, particularly Type II collagen. It is often mistakenly touted as supplying HA. Velvet antler is not an excellent oral source of HA.

Confusion reigns over which collagen products are beneficial for arthritis and other conditions. For example, native unhydrolyzed collagen is mistakenly promoted for osteoarthritis and its manufacturers have falsely claimed it is superior to hydrolyzed collagen. Ditto for another collagen product which alleges it is a superior product because it is undenatured (also called native Type II collagen), that is, it has not undergone heat or chemical treatment. The companies marketing these products cite the work of Dr. David Trentham, a Harvard professor, who is said to recommend this type of undenatured collagen supplement. The problem is, Dr. Trentham's work involved very small amounts of collagen (less than 10 milligrams) used only among patients with rheumatoid arthritis to build up oral tolerance and overcome autoimmune reaction. There is no mention of the amount of HA provided in this product, which is the key ingredient. Undenatured collagen products claim that their native collagen is not subject to high temperature or synthetic enzymes that render the supplement "less effective." Yet it is this very processing that breaks down HA into lower molecular weight fractions so it can be absorbed. Any company that does not even understand the basic science behind collagen supplementation is suspect. The native Type II collagen has a high molecular weight and it has only been shown to be appropriate in very low doses to develop oral tolerance for the treatment of rheumatoid arthritis (not osteoarthritis) only.

Autoimmune Inc., attempted but failed to achieve FDA approval for its ColloralTM collagen product as a prescription pharmaceutical drug when it failed to show improvement on morning stiffness among rheumatoid arthritis patients. It is now licensed as a food supplement under the brand name UCII, undenatured Type II collagen by Interhealth. It is derived from skin and bones of cattle and large doses could trigger an immune response in sensitive individuals. UCII is only intended for use among rheumatoid arthritis sufferers.

Chondroitin sulfate and glucosamine sulfate are also commonly consumed as food supplements, usually for the treatment of osteoarthritis. Absorption of chondroitin sulfate is about 10-15% versus 90-98% for glucosamine. However, chondroitin sulfate has been found to be superior in clinical studies. The common dosage recommendations are 1200 milligrams of glucosamine sulfate and 800 milligrams of chondroitin sulfate daily.

Abnormal levels of HA have been reported in the following conditions:
• Calcified heart valves (mitral valve)
• Osteoarthritis
• Rheumatoid arthritis
• Glaucoma
• Keratoconus
• Floaters of the eyes
• Retinal detachment
• TMJ problems
• Premature aging syndromes, such as progeria, Ehlers-Danlos syndrome
• Sun aged skin
• Premature wrinkled skin (acrogeria)
• Vocal cord problems
• Connective tissue disorders like Marfan and Stickler syndromes or Osteogenesis imperfecta

CHAPTER ELEVEN

Summary and Conclusions

Much is being learned about hyaluronic acid, this unusual molecule that holds water in the human body.

HA AND AGING

With advancing years, or disease, there may be a net daily loss of HA in body tissues. Around age 60 adults need to supplement HA production in the body by about 150 milligrams of oral HA supplement along with chondroitin sulfate.

NEED FOR HYDRATION WITH HA SUPPLEMENTS

HA is a hydrated gel, that is, it is filled with H2O. Think of HA is a chain of small pillows filled with water. One of the reasons why consumers may find that supplementation with HA, chondroitin sulfate and glucosamine sulfate take many weeks before relief from painful symptoms of arthritis is achieved is because of the lack of hydration. Because the HA molecule can hold up to 10,000 times its original volume in water, the provision of oral HA supplements should be accompanied by increased water consumption, at least four glasses of water daily. Eat grapes, melons and other water-rich foods. While many health authorities recommend increased daily consumption of water, their advice usually results in increased trips to the bathroom. The net gain is zero since the body usually controls hydration very tightly. Pure (non-chlorinated) sources of water, such as bottled or filtered water, are recommended. This obvious recommendation has apparently been overlooked by medical authorities.

FIBROSING DISEASES

This book reveals natural therapies for fibrosing diseases. Taurine and arginine are amino acids that can be consumed as dietary supplements for patients with fibrosing diseases, such as lung fibrosis and congestive heart failure.

HA AND CANCER THERAPY

The use of HA in the field of cancer therapy is intriguing because of its striking demonstrated ability to subdue cancers in animals. It is interesting to note that most cancer patients develop reduced oral intake of fluids or dehydration just before death. [Annals Oncology 10: 1255-58, 1999] This is no surprise since cancer may be destroying the HA in the body.

LETTER FROM A USER OF ORAL HYALURONIC ACID (BIOCELL COLLAGEN II™)

"My wife and I were driving back from Dallas, TX to our home in Houston, TX when we heard a commercial on one of the local Dallas radio stations touting your Ultimate H.A. Formula and decided to try it out. We received our order about three weeks later and have been taking the capsules for a month now. We have only been taking two capsules each daily and something is really going on!

My wife is a receptionist for one of the schools in our district and has just recently began getting questions on what she is doing to be so healthy looking from many of her coworkers and the children's parents coming in.

I have noticed her appearance change gradually over the last month but others we haven't seen for a while can't get over the transition of her looks. My wife is 49 years old and looks better now than most women 10 to 15 years her junior! Her skin as well as mine is very smooth and soft to the touch now and I'm 51 years old. Lines in our faces have all but disappeared and we have a much healthier look in our faces as well as the rest of our body.

I must admit I had reservations about whether your product would really work and do what the claims said it would do, but I'm a believer now and my wife and I are both very satisfied with your product.

KE
Houston, TX

Dietary factors that help to preserve HA also appear to cause cancer cells to die off in a normal fashion (bioflavonoids like quercetin, IP6 rice bran extract, Echinacea). Cells send signals that encourage programmed cell death (apoptosis) or growth (mitosis).

Cancer is when there is an irregularity in cell turnover rates. The genes that suppress tumors are weakened and the genes that activate tumors (oncogenes) become dominant. Cancer cells are immortal cells. They do not mature and die off in a normal fashion (apoptosis). Various dietary components that help preserve HA may also help to induce apoptosis in a gradual manner. For example, the bioflavonoid quercetin in red onions induces apoptosis. [Zhongguo Yao Li Xue Bao 18: 280-83, 1997] Polyphenols in tea leaves induce apoptosis. [Cancer Letters 121: 163-67, 1997] Depriving tumor cells of iron can induce apoptosis. [FEBS Letters 350: 139-42, 1994]

Paradoxically, riboflavin, a B vitamin, has been shown to induce apoptosis by virtue of its ability to degrade HA. [Investigative Ophthalmology 40: 911-19, 1999] This dual nature of HA should not remain a puzzle. For adults who want to prevent cancer, or others who want to treat existing tumors, the best advice is to utilize short, low-molecular weight HA combined with metal chelators to preserve the HA barrier that surrounds living cells. HA not only serves as a barrier against cancer, but also against infection.

Hyaluronidase causes HA to lose its viscosity, like Jello turning to water, and germs can spread. A similar mechanism occurs in the spread of tumors. [Am Journal Veterinary Research 50: 2060-63, 1989]

THE MALE BIRTH CONTROL PILL

Another striking discovery in HA-related research is the ability to utilize a natural approach to male contraception. The revelation that hyaluronidase, the enzyme that breaks down HA, is needed to successfully fertilize the female egg (ovum) by sperm, is instructive. Heavy use of hyaluronidase inhibitors by males and females, such as quercetin, Echinacea, grape seed extract, green tea, and other bioflavonoids, may significantly reduce the odds of successful conception.

EXCESS RIBOFLAVIN AND AGING

Another revelation is the role of riboflavin (vitamin B2) in human health. Excessive riboflavin can be troublesome, and many vitamin pills provide hundreds of times more vitamin B2 than recommended daily levels of consumption. Researchers in France report that exposure to solar ultraviolet light combined with excessive riboflavin can "damage HA, causing inflammation and accelerated aging in organs and tissues that are permeable to light." [Free Radical Biology Medicine 22: 1139-44, 1997] Note that excessive riboflavin accelerates aging, not just specific diseases or the breakdown of certain tissues. High-dose riboflavin supplements (more than 10 milligrams) should be avoided.

RIBOFLAVIN AND ACETAMINOPHEN

Riboflavin may have something to do with toxic liver problems brought on by the use of acetaminophen pain relievers. Acetaminophen (Tylenol) is a commonly-used pain reliever. The primary drawback of acetaminophen is that it may produce liver toxicity that can result in death or the need for a liver transplant. Over 70,000 cases of acetaminophen poisoning are reported annually in the USA. In an animal test, rodents completely deprived of dietary riboflavin exhibited complete protection against acetaminophen toxicity. [Drug Nutrient Interactions 2; 183-91, 1983] The combination of high-dose riboflavin, which could occur among individuals taking some high-dose B vitamin pills, along with acetaminophen could have serious undesirable consequences.

EXCESS HA

While much can be said for HA supplementation in the diet, particularly after age 60 when most adults begin to experience overt signs of aging such as stiff joints, wrinkles and diminished eyesight, there are also many conditions where excessive HA accumulates in localized tissues, such as the heart, lung and bowel in states of disease. [Journal Internal Medicine 242: 49-55, 1997] HA accumulates in tissues that are undergoing healing. It is unlikely that low-molecular weight oral HA supplements will affect these localized conditions.

BEE VENOM THERAPY

Venom from insects, fish or snakes contains hyaluronidase, the enzyme that breaks down HA. Venom may be harmful or beneficial.

Venom has been used by the Chinese to treat certain health problems. A British Broadcasting Company news report tells the story of Joe de Casa, a 61-year old had arthritis in his thumbs. He was bitten by an adder snake on the hand while gardening. His arthritis symptoms in the bitten hand disappeared for a period of weeks. [BBC News May 5, 2002] Another report shows that patients

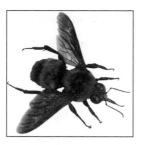

Bee venom may actually have bona fide therapeutic applications for the treatment of arthritis. The bee venom can be applied orally or topically.

who undergo acupuncture and who also apply bee venom to the treatment site appear to experience greater pain relief than acupuncture-only treated patients. [American Journal Chinese Medicine 29: 187-99, 2001] Other studies confirm that bee venom may be helpful, particularly for rheumatoid arthritis. [Acupuncture Electrotherapy Research 26: 59-68, 2001; Pain 90: 271-80, 2001] Bee venom is alleged to excite the production of cortisol, a natural steroidal hormone. Steroids drugs are used to treat arthritis.

On the other hand, a study of beekeepers in Spain shows that more than half report episodes of arthritis in their hands from bee stings at the time of honey collection. Maybe a little bit of bee venom is desirable, but too much is harmful. [Journal Rheumatology 26: 2684-90, 1999]

Bee venom therapy is often mislabeled as medical quackery. Some companies sell bee venom rub and bee venom capsules which are said to increase the body's production of cortisol, a steroidal hormone secreted from the adrenal glands. Steroid drugs are employed in arthritis treatment to reduce pain and inflammation. Possibly bee venom naturally stimulates steroids that inhibit pain and inflammation. Bee venom by virtue of its hyaluronidase content may be useful in treating lymphedema (leg swelling) often associated with cancer treatment, and morning joint stiffness in rheumatoid arthritis.

Blocking hyaluronidase may also be helpful. For example, Echinacea is an herb that traditionally has been used to treat snake bite. Echinacea blocks the spread of snake venom by inhibiting the hyaluronidase enzyme. Along with a rubber suction cup to remove venom from a snake bite, every snake bite kit ought to include Echinacea capsules which should be taken orally immediately following a bite.

HA: POTENTIAL SIDE EFFECTS

There are some potential side effects from taking oral HA supplements. Excessive HA, which may accumulate during healing, traps water and could result in swelling. [Journal Biological Chemistry 277: 4593-96, 2002] Reports that HA may thicken the lymph fluid emphasizes the use of low-molecular weight oral HA supplements and the avoidance of HA supplements among patients with lymphedema (leg swelling).

Similarly, because of HA's ability to thicken fluids such as the bile, supplemental HA should not be consumed by patients with obstructed or narrow bile ducts (primary sclerosing cholangitis). HA increases the viscosity of blood and lymph fluid. Chondroitin sulfate increases the viscosity of HA even though chondroitin sulfate is not very viscous itself. [Biochim Biopohys Acta 1380: 1-9, 1998] It's theoretically possible that oral HA would increase the viscosity of the blood and can possibly elevate blood pressure, though excess HA is being dumped into the blood circulation in rheumatoid arthritis and other diseases without an observed effect upon blood pressure.

CHAPTER TWELVE

Other Anti-aging Strategies

Readers should be urged to learn beyond HA in their quest to remain young.

For example, Dr. Bruce Ames and his associates at the University of California, Berkeley, reports an astounding breakthrough in age reversal. They found that two food supplements commonly sold in health food stores put the spark back into the life of aging rats.

Animals whose diet was supplemented with alpha lipoic acid, a sulfur compound naturally found in the body, and acetyl L carnitine, an amino acid also found in the body's cells, profoundly reversed memory loss and age-related energy decline. Activity levels improved so much in these rats that it was equivalent to a 75-80 year old person becoming middle-aged once again, said the researchers. [Proceeding National Academy Sciences 99: 1870-75, 2002; 99: 1876-78, 2002 and 99: 3356,-61, 2002]

For humans, about 1500 milligrams of acetyl L-carnitine and 200 milligrams of alpha lipoic acid would

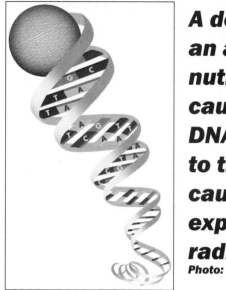

A deficiency of an array of nutrients can cause injury to DNA equivalent to the damage caused by exposure to radiation.
Photo: DOEGenomestoLife.org

be recommended on a daily basis, particularly older adults.

Another remarkable study reveals for the first time how DNA repairs itself. This genetic material is strung out on a line making up a chromosome. Think of the DNA strand, which holds what are called nucleotides (amino acids attached to sugar molecule) as a wash line held at each end of two poles. If the DNA strand breaks at one end, enzymes are produced which carefully repair the break and link up the DNA strand to its anchor. But if both ends of the DNA strand are broken, what is called a double-DNA strand break, that is serious trouble. Up till recently scientists didn't even know how DNA could repair itself when both ends break. Now they know.

The molecule that facilitates double-strand DNA repair is called phytic acid (IP6), a component of whole grains and seeds. [Cell 102: 721-29, 2000] Known as a mineral chelator, IP6 is known to have remarkable anti-aging qualities. Without IP6 the worst type of DNA damage cannot be repaired.

Aging doesn't begin in the human body till after full growth is attained. Thereafter there is an accumulation of minerals, particularly iron and copper, which slowly rust out living tissues. After age 18 the human body accumulates about 1 milligram of excess iron per day of life.

Females, being the baby carriers of life, must be protected from disease so they dump their excess iron once a month in the process of menstruation and avoid overmineralization. Females have half the iron levels of males and half the diabetes, heart disease, cancer and rate of infections. Females also universally outlive males. Once women undergo a hysterectomy or begin menopause and no longer have a monthly cycle, they begin to experience the same rate of disease as males.

The periodic donation of blood, which carries 80 percent of the iron in the body, reduces the incidence of disease and prolongs life. The removal (chelation) of excessive metals, such as iron, copper, mercury and others, would serve to prolong life and reverse aging changes. Phytic acid, known as IP6 in health food stores, is a potent mineral chelator, safer, more effective and economical than EDTA chelation therapy performed in a doctor's office.

A course of 1600-3600 milligrams of IP6 rice bran extract, taken with water only on an empty stomach, will remove excessive minerals from the body (chelation). A 1 to 3-month program using IP6 should serve to reverse many of the effects of aging due to toxic metal overload. [The Iron Time Bomb, Here & Now Books, Bill Sardi, 2000] IP6 chelation therapy removes calcium deposits from the blood vessels, kidneys and heart valves (mitral valve), and removes toxic heavy metals like cadmium, lead and mercury, from the brain.

Aging in the brain is of great concern. Memory loss begins in middle age and continues on throughout life. The number of aged adults with Alzheimer's disease is growing. Alzheimer's disease is associated with tangled plaques in the brain called beta amyloid. Is there anything that could reverse aging changes in the brain?

Researchers added ferulic acid, an antioxidant found in plants like ginkgo biloba, to the diet of mice. Then researchers injected beta amyloid plaque material into the brain of these animals. Mice that did not receive

Alzheimer's disease is associated with tangled plaques in the brain called beta amyloid. Ferulic acid, a component of ginkgo biloba, counters the adverse effects of beta amyloid and has been shown to prevent memory loss in animals injected with beta amyloid.

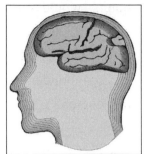

ferulic acid exhibited a decline in their ability to navigate a maze. But the animals given ferulic acid actually improved their memory and navigation scores. [British Journal Pharmacology 133: 89-96, 2001]

Another natural compound, derived from Chinese club moss, called huperzine A, is also gaining attention for its ability to reverse memory loss in humans. Huperzine A was traditionally used to treat fevers and inflammation in Chinese medicine. But it was observed that it also aided memory. [Acta Medicine 41: 155-57, 1998] In one study huperzine A was found to be more effective in animals than tacrine, a drug used to treat Alzheimer's disease. [Zhongguo Yao Li Xue Bao 19; 27-30, 1998] Huperzine A works by helping the brain to retain adequate acetycholine levels. Acetycholine is the memory molecule in the brain. [Current Medical Chemistry 7: 355-74, 2000]

Supplementation with 200 micrograms of huperzine A daily is safe and may be helpful in reversing memory decline in older adults. [Zhongguo Yao Li Xue bao 20: 486-90, 1999] Just 100 micrograms daily of huperzine A has been shown to improve learning performance among school children. [Zhongguo Yao Li Xue Bao 20: 601-03, 1999] Huperzine A was even demonstrated to improve memory after an amnesia-inducing drug was given to animals. [European Journal Pharmacology 433: 151-56, 2001]

Think of what has been shared in this book. The ravages of human aging can be potentially reversed. Humans can re-grow hair, regain flexibility of youth, recoup sharp eyesight, redeem wrinkled skin, and renew their body, as well as protect against cancer. Hyaluronic acid is a molecule that must not be ignored any longer.

SUPPLEMENT PROGRAM TO REVERSE AGING

Slowing down the aging process and reversing are two different things. A few decades back Denham Harman proposed that oxygen free radicals, the primary rusting agents of the body, promote disease and accelerate aging. The use of antioxidant vitamins which exceed the daily recommendations published by government health authorities may be beneficial in regards to slowing the aging process. Vitamin C, vitamin E, selenium and bioflavonoids comprise a long list of natural antioxidants that protect the tissues in the body from withering over time. But now we have evidence that aging can not only be slowed, it can be reversed, with hyaluronic acid, chondroitin sulfate and any array of other readily available food supplements. An age-reversal supplement regimen might look something like this.

1. Supplement a diet rich in fresh fruits and vegetables with herbs, vitamins and other nutrients that help to maintain HA. These include Echinacea, milk thistle, vitamin C, bioflavonoids from citrus, grapes and berries, and IP6 rice bran extract.

2. Replace lost HA with oral hyaluronic food supplements, at least 150 milligrams a day of HA. The best designed HA food supplement available today is Biocell Collagen II which includes Type II collagen, chondroitin sulfate and 50 full milligrams of HA per capsule.

3. Avoid or minimize factors that are known to trigger the production of hyaluronidase, the enzyme that breaks down HA. The list includes excessive solar ultraviolet radiation, any forms of ionizing radiation (xray, gamma ray), excessive vitamin B2 riboflavin supplementation (beyond 10 milligrams per day), and any supplemental iron for full-grown males, postmenopausal females or women who have undergone early hysterectomy.

4.   If over age 60, supplement the diet with 1500 milligrams of acetyl L-carnitine and 200 milligrams of alpha lipoic acid.

5.   Take vitamin C to maintain collagen. Preferably 2000 milligrams or more per day. Preferred forms of vitamin C are the buffered mineral ascorbates.

6.   If concerned over failing memory or mental acuity, try ginkgo biloba, about 240 milligrams, and/or huperzine A, about 150-200 micrograms, per day.

7.   Remove excess minerals that have built up in the body. IP6 rice bran extract, 1600-3600 milligrams, taken on a daily basis with water only on an empty stomach, effectively removes excessive minerals from the blood vessels, liver, kidneys, brain and other tissues.

8.   Take a good multivitamin. It is the cheapest health insurance you can buy. Dr. Bruce Ames of the University of California, Berkeley, reports that deficiencies of vitamin B6, niacin, vitamin C, vitamin E, iron or zinc mimics radiation in damaging DNA by causing single or double-strand breaks in DNA. Deficiencies of these nutrients ranges from 2 to 20 percent in the US population. Approximately 10 percent of US adults don't consume sufficient amounts of folic acid to prevent chromosome breaks. The quarter of the

Dr. Bruce Ames of the University of California, Berkeley, reports that deficiencies of vitamin B6, niacin, vitamin C, vitamin E, iron or zinc mimics radiation damaged DNA by causing single or double-strand breaks in DNA.

population that consumes the lowest amount of fresh fruits and vegetables has about double the cancer rate compared to adults who consume 5-7 servings of fresh plant foods daily. [Mutation Research 475: 7-20, 2001]

9.   Drink clean, purified water. The human body has a fine-tuned mechanism to control hydration. Most of the water humans consume is obtained from foods. The addition of two to four glasses of water a day will suffice for most adults. With chronic or acute disease or pain, four to eight glasses of water a day is recommended. The water should be free of chlorine which increases the risk of kidney and bladder cancer. Some 5000 cases of bladder cancer and 8000 cases of rectal cancer occur annually that are attributed to chlorination of water. [Environmental Health Perspectives 103: 225-31, 1995] Adults taking HA supplements need to drink more water to obtain the full health benefits of this molecule.

Addendum

Vitamin C—The Long-Life Vitamin

Because of vitamin C's important role in the production of collagen, and its unusual ability to lengthen the human life span, this special addendum has been added to the book.

Collagen and HA are important partners. Collagen can be likened to the mortar between bricks (living cells) and HA is the moisturizing agent that keeps the collagen from cracking and drying out. HA does not help to build collagen, vitamin C does that along with bioflavonoids.

Vitamin C has a dual personality. It is both an antioxidant (anti-rusting agent) and a pro-oxidant (indirectly promotes rusting in the body). By donating an electron, vitamin C can help to protect the oxidation of vitamin E. It also reinvigorates glutathione, another major antioxidant in the body, through the same electron donor process. Vitamin C is also a hyaluronidase inhibitor. So this vitamin helps to build collagen and prevent the breakdown of HA.

At the same time, vitamin C may alter the form of iron in the body from $Fe3+$ to $Fe2+$. This makes it possible for

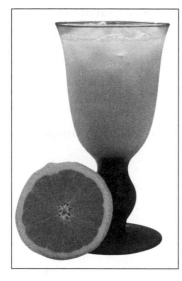

Vitamin C is the only vitamin repeatedly proven to increase the human lifespan when taken in doses that exceed dietary levels of this vitamin.

iron to become a rusting agent in the body as it detaches from proteins that normally bind to iron to keep it under control. Vitamin C may stimulate collagen production via its ability to induce lipid peroxidation. So vitamin C plays both roles, as an antioxidant which preserves collagen and oxidant to boost collagen production. It's a self-rebuilding process. Vitamin C is at the crux of the self-regenerating nature of living tissues. [Medical Hypotheses 2: 154-63, 1976]

In a perfect state of health there is no free, unbound iron in the blood circulation. But in disease, free iron is detectable and it accumulates at the site of inflammation, such as arthritic joints, tumors, and wounds. It is believed the iron accumulates at these sites in order to kill off any unfriendly organisms. However, free iron can accumulate in such a rapid and concentrated manner as to cause most of the tissue damage in disease states.

In animals that are iron overloaded, vitamin C appears to promote oxidation by releasing iron from binding proteins, but not in animals that are not iron overloaded. [British Journal Nutrition 85: 681-87, 2001]

The argument is that HA is broken down by vitamin C and thus high-dose vitamin C may be deleterious. However, in studies conducted in Germany, while it was found that ascorbic acid induces degradation of HA, this reaction is increased when iron is present. Iron-binders (chelators) completely abolish the breakdown of HA by vitamin C. [Free Radical Research Communications 3: 85-92, 1987]

It is well established that vitamin C promotes collagen formation. For example, high-dose vitamin C is very helpful to people who don't produce enough collagen and have "rubber-man syndrome" (Ehlers-Danlos syndrome).

Vitamin C stimulates collagen formation in skin fibroblast cells but does not have an effect upon HA. [Eur J Biochem 173: 679, 1988] In other studies, vitamin C has actually been shown to reduce HA production in skin. [J Cell Sci 64: 245-54, 1983] It does this by depolymerizing HA (unzipping the molecular bonds that hold HA molecules together) via its conversion of iron from Fe3+ to Fe2+. Fortunately, iron chelators halt the degradation. [Journal Inorganic Biochemistry 14: 127-34, 1981] The lesson here is clear. Vitamin C does not promote oxidation (rusting) unless free iron is available. The body makes some of its own iron-binding proteins in the liver (albumin, ferritin, transferrin, lactoferrin) but also utilizes dietary-acquired iron-binders such as bioflavonoids from citrus, grapes and berries, and phytic acid (IP6) from seeds and whole grains.

Except for a few species of monkeys, bats and guinea pigs, most animals produce their own vitamin C by converting circulating sugars into ascorbic acid.

NATURAL VITAMIN C

In stores commercial brands vitamin C are provided in two forms. One is plain ascorbic acid. This is generally not how vitamin C is provided in nature. In nature it is usually accompanied by a bioflavonoid pigment or a mineral. Mineral ascorbates, or what is called buffered vitamin C, is the more stable form and should be accompanied by a plentiful amount of bioflavonoids. Various products are available in health food stores.

VITAMIN C: PRODUCED NATURALLY BY ANIMALS

It is important to note here that vitamin C is produced naturally by most animals. The form of vitamin C produced by animals IS mineral ascorbate, that is, sodium ascorbate, calcium ascorbate, magnesium ascorbate, manganese ascorbate. The minerals and vitamin C are delivered together.

Except for a few species of monkeys, bats and guinea pigs, most animals produce their own vitamin C by converting circulating sugars into ascorbic acid. For example, an animal about the same size as a human, like a 160-pound goat, makes about 13,000 mg of vitamin C per day and more under stress.

Due to a genetic defect, humans do not produce vitamin C within the body, whereas most animals do. Most animals produce an enzyme, L-gulonolactone oxidase, which converts sugars passing through the liver or kidneys into an alkaline form of vitamin C. It is revealing to examine what happens when the gene that produces gulonolactone oxidase is intentionally altered to become dysfunctional in rats. Within a few weeks the animals lose weight, become anemic (don't produce enough red blood cells), and die. In vitamin C-deprived male rats, but not females, there is an accumulation of cholesterol in blood vessel walls. (The females have lower iron levels which minimizes the hardening of cholesterol.) There were striking abnormalities observed in the aortas of these vitamin C- deficient rats and the blood vessels throughout the body become weak. [Proceedings Natl Academy Sciences 97: 841-46, 2000]

There are four enzymes which convert glucose into vitamin C, but humans only make the first three. The gene for the gulonolactone oxidase enzyme is massively damaged and totally useless in homo sapiens.

In normal rats, vitamin C accounts for 72 percent of the antioxidant (anti-rusting) capacity in blood plasma, whereas in humans who must rely upon the diet to 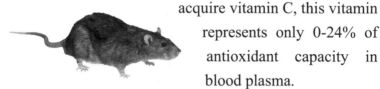 acquire vitamin C, this vitamin represents only 0-24% of antioxidant capacity in blood plasma.

The provision of the gulonolactone oxidase enzyme to guinea pigs that do not produce vitamin C increases their survivability. [Biochemistry Medical Metabolic Biology 35: 59-64, 1986] The same is true in humans. Just 300 milligrams of vitamin C per day has been shown to increase the human life span by six years, which is more than can be accomplished by exercising every day or controlling cholesterol.

A study of 11,000 Americans over 10 years revealed that individuals with the highest level of vitamin C intake, only about 300 milligrams, suffered 35 percent fewer deaths than those with the lowest intake, about 50 milligrams a day. This amounts to about 6 added years of life to those who consume higher levels of vitamin C. Since 300 milligrams of vitamin C is difficult to obtain from dietary sources alone, the primary group that exhibited increased life span were users of vitamin C supplements. [Newsweek, May 18, 1992; Epidemiology 3: 194-202, 1992] A person would have to consume five oranges a day to get 300 milligrams of vitamin C from their diet alone.

Nobel prize winner Dr. Linus Pauling suggested humans supplement their diet continually through the day to mimic what the liver would make if the gene for the gulonolactone oxidase enzyme were still active. Dr. Pauling advocated supplementation with mineral ascorbates, the same alkaline form of vitamin C the liver produces in mammals, not ascorbic acid which can sometimes be irritating to the stomach and can even eat away tooth enamel. [Pauling L, How to Live Longer and Feel Better, July 1996]

LONGEVA-C

There are additional corroborating studies that back up the idea of vitamin C supplementation and longevity.

As early as 1984 researchers knew that supplementation of drinking water with vitamin C increased the average life span of mice by as much as 20 percent. [Gerontology 30: 371-75, 1984]

A study over a 12-16-year period showed that males with the highest blood serum levels of vitamin C experienced a 57 percent drop in their risk of dying from any cause compared to males with low circulating levels of vitamin C. [American Journal Clinical Nutrition 72: 139-45, 2000]

Among men and women ages 45-79 years, just a 50 milligram increase in vitamin C consumption was able to reduce the relative all-cause mortality rate by 20 percent. [The Lancet 357: March 3, 2001]

Another study published in 2001 also confirms a 25-29 percent decreased all-cause mortality rate among adults with normal to high circulating levels of vitamin C. [J Am College Nutrition 20: June 2001]

It is interesting to note that vitamin C acts as a key agent in various models of anti-aging. Vitamin C would be a key antioxidant in the free radical theory of aging. [J Gerontology 21: 560-65, 1966] Researchers have demonstrated that vitamin C slows down telomere shortening by 52-62 percent in a controlled experiment. [Life Sciences 63: 935-48, 1998] Telomeres are the end caps of DNA that shorten with many generations and limit the number of replications of DNA.

HUMANS HAVE THE CAPACITY TO LIVE FOR HUNDREDS OF YEARS

The good news is that there is scientific evidence that humans have the capacity to lengthen their average life span by hundreds of years. The evidence for vitamin C as a key anti-aging agent is compelling and rooted in the genetic makeup of humans.

All humans are mutants. Homo sapiens, guinea pigs, monkeys, bats, some fish and many birds, do not produce their own vitamin C. The rest of the animal kingdom synthesizes its own vitamin C. For most animals, ascorbic acid is a hormone, not a dietary-acquired vitamin. Animals employ different organs to produce vitamin C. Some birds and reptiles use their kidneys and perching birds and mammals make vitamin C in their liver. [Origins 12: 96-100, 1985]

Humans once made vitamin C in their liver by the production of four enzymes which convert circulating sugars into ascorbic acid (vitamin C). Humans today only make three of the four enzymes required to convert glucose (sugar) into ascorbic acid. A progressive mutation at some time in past generations deactivated the gene for the enzyme gulonolactone oxidase and slowly as the mutation progressed the synthesis of vitamin C came to an end in humans.

Mammals that make their own vitamin C can live 8-10 times beyond their age of physical maturity. Mammals without this ability have a difficult time reaching 3-4 times. Researchers believe the reinstallation of the gulonolactone oxidase enzyme in humans would extend the lifespan to hundreds of years.

This means that humans at one time in the past, prior to this gene mutation, lived for hundreds of years. This doesn't fit with the current evolutionary scheme of biology which postulates that humans evolved from monkeys and early man lived no longer than 40 years.

WHEN DID HUMANS LIVE FOR HUNDREDS OF YEARS?

An examination of the historical records in the Holy Bible reveals that Adam was recorded to have lived for 930 years (Genesis 5:5), and Noah for 950 years

How did Adam live for more than 900 years? Early Biblical records indicate that people lived for hundreds of years. The mechanism for this longevity has now been discovered. Early humans naturally produced vitamin C, whereas modern-day humans, due to a genetic mutation, have lost this ability.

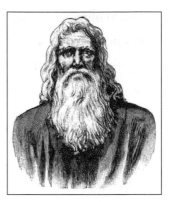

(Genesis 9:29). According to the Biblical record the human genome was severely narrowed at the time of a great worldwide flood, down to just eight members of Noah's family as gene carriers. Thereafter the human life span was recorded to slowly dissipate. After the Flood, Bible genealogies indicate Shem lived 600 years, followed by Arphaxad who lived 438 years, and through other generations on down to Abraham who lived 175 years and finally to Moses who lived 120 years (Deuteronomy 34:7). This description would fit the progressive mutation of the gulonolactone oxidase gene. Humans still house this gene, it is just defunct and called a pseudogene. Thus the Biblical genealogies may not be far-fetched fairy tales.

CAN THE ENZYME TO PRODUCE VITAMIN C BE RE-INSTALLED IN HUMANS?

What if the gulonolactone oxidase gene could somehow be re-inserted into the human genome? We know that guinea pigs lack gulonolactone oxidase. When given this enzyme by injection they are able to survive on a diet deficient in vitamin C. [J Inherit Metabolic Diseases 11: 387-96, 1988]

Scientists have taken the gulonolactone oxidase DNA from rat liver and successfully tranplanted it into the tomato genome. [Plant Biology '97, Abstract 1545] The gulonolactone oxidase gene has also been successfully transferred into a teleost fish (Oryzias latipes) via microinjection into fertilized fish eggs. [Biochem Biophys Res Commun 223: 650-53, 1996]

With all of the widely heralded prospects for gene therapy there hasn't been a peep about the feasability of inserting the gulonolactone oxidase gene into the human genome. Yet the profound impact of such a development, if successful, would obviously be monumental. Diabetes, blood vessel disease, cataracts, gallstones, to name a few age-related maladies, would be eradicated. The breakdown of collagen with advancing age would be slowed.

The world human population jumped from 1.6 to 6.1 billion in the past century, 2 billion of that growth coming since 1960, largely from improvements in sanitation, food fortification and modern medicines. [Population Reference Bureau, 2002]   Imagine the social, political and medical ramifications if humans could live for hundreds of years?

HOW MUCH VITAMIN C?

How much vitamin C should humans ingest? If you want to get all your vitamin C from foods, consumption of the recommended 5 to 7 servings of fruits and vegetables a day is likely to provide 200-250 milligrams. A mouse makes about 275 milligrams of vitamin C per day per kilogram (2.2 lbs) of body weight. If a mouse weighed 154 pounds, about the weight of a human, this would amount to about 19,250 milligrams of vitamin C per day. A 160-pound goat produces about 13,000 milligrams per day, and more under stress. A dog or cat will produce about 40 milligrams of vitamin C per kilogram of body weight per day, or the equivalent of 2800 mgs per day if these animals were about the same size as humans. So using animals as a rule of thumb, humans may benefit from consumption of anywhere from 2,000-20,000 milligrams per day. The only common side effect from high-dose vitamin C is a transient diarrhea-like buildup of water in the lower bowel.

Government health authorities recommend only about 90 milligrams of vitamin C a day for adults, but that's just the minimum amount to prevent scurvy and promote general health, not to achieve optimal health and longevity. Studies indicate the vitamin C intake for Americans is around 110 milligrams per day, but adequate vitamin C status, even with food fortification, is still not guaranteed. According to one study, about 1-2 percent of college students exhibited true deficiency and marginal deficiencies were found in an additional 12-16 percent of students. [J Am College Health 46: 209-13, 1998]

IS HIGH-DOSE VITAMIN C GENOTOXIC?

However, with all of this positive information about vitamin C, the news media recently chose to widely circulate a misleading test-tube study claiming high-dose vitamin C is toxic to DNA which could cause cancer. Researchers recommended vitamin C supplements be restricted to no more than 200 milligrams per day. This report caused the public to temporarily pause in the consumption vitamin C supplements. [Science 292: 2083-86, 2001] However, the 200-milligram limit conflicts with government health authorities who recommend consumption of 5-7 servings of fruits and vegetables per day which would likely provide more than the 200 milligram amount. Virtually all evidence from dietary studies confirms the health benefits of foods that provide high amounts of vitamin C. Another earlier study published in Nature indicated 500 milligrams of vitamin C in humans may produce damage to DNA in lymphocytes, a type of white blood cell. [Nature 392: 559, 1998] However, other studies reveal that vitamin C actually protects against DNA damage to lymphocytes but this protective effect is greatly enhanced when accompanied by bioflavonoids which usually accompany vitamin C in nature. [Am J Clin Nutrition 67: 1210-18, 1998] Bioflavonoids are plant pigments commonly found in citrus, berries, grapes and tea leaves. The better store brands of buffered vitamin C powder (mineral ascorbates) include bioflavonoids. Furthermore, five other subsequent human studies were conducted using high-dose vitamin C up to 5000 milligrams per day and could not find evidence that vitamin C induces gene mutations. [Science 293: 5537, 2001]

Then there is the aforementioned evidence from the animal kingdom where animals produce thousands of milligrams of vitamin C daily without evidence this induces gene mutations or cancer. A modern mountain gorilla living in its natural habitat, that produces no vitamin C on its own, would obtain 4,500 milligrams of vitamin C per day from native foodstuffs. [British J Nutrition 2: 341, 1949] A 15-pound howler monkey takes in 600 milligrams of vitamin C per day and an 18-pound spider monkey consumes about 744 milligrams of vitamin C per day. [Dept. Anthropology, University of Calif. Berkeley, 14th Intl Congress on Anthropological and Ethnological Sciences, July 26, 1998] There is no evidence that these levels of vitamin C from dietary sources induce any DNA mutations or cancer in these animals.

Furthermore, there are studies which reveal significant health benefits for humans who consume vitamin C in excess of the newly established 90 milligram reference daily intake. For example, human studies reveal that 300 milligrams of daily vitamin C appears to reduce the risk of blinding cataracts, an otherwise inevitable consequence of aging, by 77-83 percent. [Am J Clinical Nutrition 66: 911-16, 1997] A 500-milligram daily dose of vitamin C has been found to significantly reduce blood pressure among hypertensive patients who previously had to use prescription medications. [The Lancet 354: Dec. 11, 1995]

TOO LITTLE COLLAGEN AND HA
(RUBBER-MAN SYNDROME)

Insufficient collagen production can result is what is called "rubber-man syndrome" (Ehlers-Danlos syndrome) where the skin is easily stretchable and the skin and tendons are weak. Other signs of this syndrome are floppy ears, varicose veins, ability to hyperextend joints, reversal of spinal curvature and eye problems (retinal detachment, glaucoma, corneal tears).

Vitamin C increases the production of collagen in Ehlers-Danlos syndrome via its ability to increase levels of hysl hydroxylase, an enzyme required to produce collagen. [Archives Biochemistry Biophysics 321: 510-16, 1995] The fibroblast cells that produce HA in normally healthy individuals do not produce as much HA in patients with Elhers-Danlos syndrome.

High-dose vitamin C is very therapeutic to patients with Ehlers-Danlos syndrome. One year of 5000 mg of vitamin C per day improved wound healing, muscle strength and bleeding time. [Metabolism 36: 687-91, 1987] It was previously shown in cases of inherited collagen that the provision of 4000 milligrams of vitamin C per day improved wound healing, muscle strength and corneal diameter over a two-year period. [Journal Pediatrics 92: 378-84, 1978]

STARTING LIFE WITHOUT ENOUGH VITAMIN C

Too little vitamin C in the human diet, and thus poor collagen production, can cause problems right from birth. The lack of vitamins C and E during pregnancy can lead to premature delivery due to a rupture of the fetal membrane. Current prenatal vitamins provide less than the suggested levels to prevent this occurrence. [Am Journal Obstetrics and Gynecology 185: 5-10, 2001] Pregnant females who do not get enough vitamin

C from their diet or supplements may experience a ruptured membrane and deliver a premature baby. The fetal membrane attached to the placenta is composed of collagen. Collagen production is facilitated by vitamin C. Women who consume very little vitamin C have double the risk of a ruptured membrane. [Reuters Health, January 18, 2002]

VITAMIN C AND CANCER

In 1976 Linus Pauling reported on the use of mega-dose vitamin C among terminal cancer patients. The survival time among terminal cancer patients who did not consume supplemental vitamin C was 50 days whereas the patients who took vitamin C survived on average about 210 days. This is about a 400 percent increase in survivability, something that has never been duplicated in a clinical study using conventional cancer therapy. Some of the terminal patients who took vitamin C lived 20 times longer than those who did not take vitamin C. [Proc Natl Academy Science 73: 3685-89, 1976]

Vitamin C has many modes of action against cancer including boosting of immunity and countering the deleterious effects of nitrosamine compounds in foods (like bacon). [Proc Natl Academy Sci 87: 7245-59, 1990; Mutation Research 428: 353-61, 1999 and Nutrition & Cancer 31: 106-10, 1998] But more important is vitamin

C's role in maintaining collagen and thus inhibiting the spread or metastasis of cancer. Vitamin C along with the amino acids lysine and proline are utilized to form collagen. [Biochim Biophys Acta 675: 117-22, 1981; Yale Journal Biology Medicine 58: 553-59, 1985] In a laboratory dish vitamin C increases the production of collagen by 8 times! [Proc Natl Academy Science 78: 2879-82, 1981] This is consistent with the fact that the breakdown of the collagen matrix is required for cancer cells to invade and spread. An cancer treatment regimen should include vitamin C combined with lysine, proline and other iron-binding antioxidants such as green tea, IP6 rice bran extract or quercetin, in order to help maintain collagen and thus cement the cancer cells in place so they cannot spread.

Resources

Purity Products
139 Haven Avenue
Port Washington, New York 11050
1 888-313-7873
www.purityproducts.com
Markets ULTIMATE HA FORMULA, providing BIOCELL
COLLAGEN II™ (Type II collagen with 150 milligrams
chondroitin sulfate and 50 milligrams hyaluronic acid with
quercetin, IP6 rice bran extract and vitamin C). Low HA
molecular weight 1500-3000 Daltons. Purity Products also
offers an advanced HA formula called VITALAMAX which
provides HA in BioCell Collagen II™, marine lipid oils,
antioxidants, vitamin C, and coenzyme Q10.

Kinetic Technologies
P.O. Box 12388
Lexington, Kentucky 40583
1 877-786-9882
www.kinetictech.net
Markets NU-LIFE hyaluronic acid formula providing 20
milligrams of HA per capsule from a synthetic source; also
markets HA products for veterinary use.

Soft Gel Technologies, Inc.
6982 Bandini Boulevard
Los Angeles, California 90040
1 800-360-SGTI
www.soft-gel.com
Markets INJUV hyaluronic acid, 9 milligrams per capsule
from rooster comb source.

Honeybee Therapy, LLC
P.O. Box 671 Big Horn, WY 82833
Toll free 1-866-289-9233, in Wyoming
1-866-289-9233
1-307-673-5917
Website: www.honeybeetherapy.com
E-mail: buzz@honeybeetherapy.com
Provides honey bee venom as topical treatment for aches and
pains.

Index

P

Q

R

S

T

U

—NOTES—

—NOTES—

—NOTES—

—NOTES—

—NOTES—

—NOTES—